Praise for *Look at Me, I'm Talking to You!*

"As a Naturopathic Doctor, I read many books, most of which are technically orientated. Although I was aware of most observable deficiency symptoms presented in this book, Bob made them easier to recognize for the lay person. I heartily recommend it to moms and dads and those of us in this industry."

—Robert David Kantor, N.D.

"The language of the human body is as eloquent as it is accurate. How can we expect the conscious mind alone to cope with the extraordinarily complex language of this beautiful organism when we are able to use only a small fraction of it? Yet we turn to the brilliantly educated healthcare industry for answers and prescriptions, a terrible path that ultimately leads us to pain and suffering. If Bob Weiss' compelling little book stands for anything, it is a curriculum for the most important thing we, each of us, can learn to better understand ourselves and each other, just as he did so well during an impressive career as a health store owner, and that is to listen."

—Stephen Quinto, CEO, Natural-Immunogenics Corp.

"During the 20 years of practicing medicine in both Internal Medicine and Emergency Medicine, I have realized how much can be learned during the physical examination just by simple observation. It is a skill we are taught early on in training, but truly takes years to develop. Bob Weiss has clearly developed that skill. His book, *Look at Me,* is entertaining and compelling reading regarding the importance of observation and its application to our nutritional health and vitamin deficiencies. Each story has essential information regarding various disease processes and their possible therapies. The information contained in this book will help healthcare professionals as well as lay people in countless ways. I applaud Bob Weiss for his success in writing this book."

—Edward Nichols, M.D.

"I've known Bob for 26 years, the life of my practice. I have treated his family and he has treated mine. It's about time he wrote this book, he has been in the trenches with sick people for many years. He ***knows.***"

—Rodger Phillips, D.C.

"As a practicing holistic professional, I see daily, the misery that so many people endure due to the lack of this information. Fatigue, headaches, frequent illness and pain are generally accepted as "life" due to lack of information and the fact that symptoms of dis-ease are, sadly, common enough to be considered normal. Life is meant to be lived joyfully. I believe everyone who wants to live a rich, happy life should read this book." —Linda Chenaur, D.C.

"Despite all the talk about vitamins today, few people actually know what they are and why they are so important. *Look at Me* is unique in that it is a textbook in short story form. These stories are both fun and easy to read, and while doing so, I was learning how to identify nutritional deficiencies."

—Sindy Celmer, N.C.

"We study to learn, but how many times have you read a book where you enjoyed reading it while learning at the same time? I read it once, and then I read it again. *Look at Me* is now required reading for all of our employees."

—Caroline Wong, store owner

LOOK AT ME I'M TALKING TO YOU!

1/3/08
CINDY,
THANKS FOR BEING YOU!
Bob Weiss

Look At Me I'm Talking To You!

Bob Weiss

The Cannon Corps • Bakersfield, CA

Published by: The Cannon Corps
12400 Trinity River Dr.
Bakersfield, CA 93312, USA
www.VitaminStories.com

LOOK AT ME, I'M TALKING TO YOU!
Bob Weiss

ISBN: 0-9778589-0-1

Book Design by Pamela Terry, Opus 1 Design
Editor: Brookes Nohlgren, Books by Brookes

Printed in United States of America

Dedication

To Pat,
my partner and dear wife of over 51 years.

To our two daughters,
Peggy and Cathy, and
our son, Bob,

To Maureen,
who did the initial editing of grammar and punctuation, but mostly gave me the encouragement to continue on with this quest.

To the many who worked side-by-side with us in our retail stores. We were blessed to have them as co-workers: Berti, Sindy, Bette, Jenni, Joani, John, Tricia, Mike, Ron, Tom, Steve, Roger, Milan, Sheila, Geneva, Heather, Betty, Karen, Phyllis, Gini, Eddie, Traci, Matt, Maile, Rick, Donna, Kathleen, Gayle…

To the specialists who helped in the production of the book:
Pam, Brookes, Helen, and Laren.

But mostly, to you, the customer
who made these stories possible through your belief in yourself and the role good nutrition plays in one's well-being.

About The Author

Bob Weiss started in the vitamin industry in 1975, then opened his first retail store, "Here's to Your Health," in Newhall, California, in 1977. In time, he was operating four stores and a nationwide mail-order business.

Health product wholesalers know him as a savvy business person who, despite frequent threats of being run out of business by larger chain stores, was able to continue the growth and expansion of his business. Bob knew how to negotiate the best prices and pass those savings on to his customers, and he kept his finger on the pulse of the industry so that his stores were stocked full with the basics as well as the cutting-edge products. In order to provide the best supplements, Bob formed his own line of products that earned national recognition.

But Bob's business ability took second seat to his customers, who constantly benefited from his passion for helping people improve their health through nutritional supplements. He was known by his customers to possess a keen ability to "read" people, both those he knew and strangers entering the store for the first time. Whether by looking into their eyes, or touching their hands during a greeting, Bob could detect their nutritional needs. Those he helped returned the favor by sharing their stories of how their health and their lives were changed by his counsel. Many asked him to tell them how he knew so much about them through just a glance.

Over the years, he began to recognize that his ability was unique, but that it could be taught. Armed with that knowledge, he recorded his experiences with a vision to help retail stores owners, nutritional consultants, and individuals learn the techniques for understanding how to interpret the body's signs.

This book has been a 30-year project for Bob, starting with the first success story shared by a customer and, eventually, ending up on paper after his retirement in 2005.

For free updates and other beneficial health infomation
from Bob, register at *VitaminStories.com*

Disclaimer

The information contained in this book is presented for general education purposes only. It is not intended to be a substitute for specific medical advice, nor in place of a physician or qualified health care practitioner. It is designed for use in conjunction with the services provided by physicians practicing, or receptive to, natural medicine.

In reading this book, one may be tempted to make his own diagnosis and to render his own treatment as indicated by some of the examples as mentioned in this book. This could be unfortunate, because one might go astray in his attempt at diagnosing his own condition. Readers are strongly urged to develop a good relationship with a physician knowledgeable in the art and science of natural and preventive medicine such as a naturopathic physician. Once established, then while talking over his problem with the doctor, he might mention the things he has gained from reading these methods of recognizing possible deficiency of a nutrient.

We must remember that every individual's response to vitamins, minerals, herbs, and other nutritional therapies is greatly different, depending on his specific condition, individual requirements and needs, age, health stature, his ability to assimilate nutrients, his emotional health, etc., etc.

change into a customer's hand, I touch the palm and then drag my fingers across the hand and up to the fingertips. I do it quickly and ever-so-lightly but enough to determine if a deficiency exists. I touch the hand to see if it is moist or clammy. I feel the fingers for warmth or coldness. No one has ever suspected this swift gesture or my intentions.

As for the woman who just entered my store, if her hand or fingers had been cold, I would look to see if she had dry hair or brittle fingernails. If so, I would ask her additional questions relevant to a deficiency of iodine and vitamin A. Eventually, my questioning might lead me to the conclusion that she was exhibiting symptoms of a low thyroid condition, or hypothyroidism. If her hand had been moist, I would ask her if she experienced headaches, dizziness upon arising, or if her family had a history of blood sugar problems, including diabetes, hypoglycemia, or alcoholism. A *yes* answer to any of these questions would lead me to corresponding questions. I would keep searching for the underlying cause of her ailment. Moreover, I would presume that, as a female, her problem might be associated with menstruation or, depending on her age, pre-menopause or menopause. Through tactful questioning, I could easily obtain this information.

Now that she and I are in close proximity, I am able to look for other symptoms. Does she have nervous twitches? Is she squinting? Are her eyes bloodshot or does she have dark circles under them? Are there bags under or around her eyes? The nose, teeth, mouth, ears, lips, and even behaviors such as yawning or swallowing are readily observed and may indicate possible deficiencies. Does she have an impaired walk? What is the condition of her skin? Is she sniffling, sneezing, or coughing? Does she appear to have a weight problem? All of these are telltale signs of a possible nutrient deficiency.

This is how I read my customers. This is how they reveal to me, through their body language, what might be the underlying cause of their problem. I am able to recognize over fifty symptoms of the deficiency of a vitamin, mineral, hormonal condition, and digestive enzyme. These bodily signals will be explained in the book.

Other symptoms are not so obvious but can be determined through conversation and in-depth questioning. For example, a coated tongue, excessive upper or lower gas, night blindness, bleeding gums, menstrual cramping, or constipation, although not obvious, can be discovered through questioning. To save time, I use a body language questionnaire that asks almost 300 questions regarding symptoms of nutritional deficiencies. From the computerized results of this questionnaire, a client can ascertain his or her nutritional insufficiencies.

Besides "reading" a client's symptoms, having knowledge of nutrients themselves is essential in determining a client's needs. Most of us know that leg cramps are most always associated with a calcium deficiency. Even the medical profession accepts this theory and usually prescribes calcium accordingly. But one should also suspect a deficiency of potassium, vitamin E, magnesium, or vitamin B-6. Improper digestion and assimilation should also be considered. If these other nutrients are not taken into consideration and the prescribed calcium doesn't work, the usual result is the prescribing of a painkiller or sedative.

When someone asks me what to take for leg cramps, I never prescribe anything; after all, I am not a doctor. I do, however, ask questions relating to specific nutrients. By selectively asking questions relevant to each of these nutrients, I can usually determine which nutritional deficiency is the probable cause. I then keep a scorecard in my head—calcium had one *yes*, magnesium had one *yes*, B-6 did not have a *yes* (except the leg cramps), and potassium had four *yes* answers. What conclusion can be reached? The accumulation of *yes* answers points to a deficiency of potassium, not calcium. This investigative procedure is successful in the majority of cases, and it is fun and rewarding.

Over the years, many customers have thanked me for correcting their various illnesses, in particular, arthritis. They describe their medically diagnosed arthritic condition as an ache or pain in the joints or other parts of the body. I do not treat any specific ailment because I am not a doctor. In fact, I take the medical diagnosis only briefly into account and then ask nutrient related questions relevant to the symptoms. Through this in-depth questioning, I find that most of these clients are actually deficient in one or more minerals, and their symptoms only mimic arthritis. By taking the proper supplements, which were lacking in their diet, they are able to correct their nutritional deficiencies, and the symptoms disappear, as does their mis-diagnosed arthritis.

If after an adequate intake of vitamin or mineral supplementation the symptoms persist, a condition other than a nutritional deficiency may exist. I always advise my client to get professional help, preferably from a medical doctor who is nutritionally oriented. The symptoms I look for and/or see do not alone prove an existing nutritional deficiency; such symptoms may be caused by a great number of conditions or functional disorders.

A clarification must be made here about identifying a single nutritional deficiency. A deficiency of a single vitamin is highly unlikely. If someone is deficient in a particular vitamin, for instance, riboflavin, or vitamin B-2, one could also assume that the person is most likely deficient in other unknown vitamins as well. Typically, I suggest that my client take the nutrient that is most obviously deficient and, to ensure that all nutrients are included, a multiple vitamin.

Look at Me, I'm Talking to You! is for anyone who is interested in a nutritional approach to helping the body heal itself.

This book is for every health food store owner, who should not only read it, of course, but also study it and adopt its principles. You will learn over fifty observable symptoms of possible nutrient deficiency. Learning what these are and how to correct them through supplementation will enhance your sales tremendously. Your knowledge will also increase your customers' confidence both in you and the vitamin industry. This increased confidence comes from the positive results the customer experiences. Your customers will tell others, and so on.

This book is also for the health food store employee, who should also read it and adopt its principles. By reading the stories in this book and noticing correspondences between symptoms and the nutritional deficiencies, you will more readily glean needed information than you would by studying those thick, multi-paged health manuals. Your confidence will also increase as you learn what questions to ask and then determine, through the customer's answers, what the nutrient needs are.

Most of all, this book is for you, the everyday person. This book is written for the mom who is also the doctor, pharmacist, nurse, and dietician for her family, along with the multitude of other jobs a mom must do. You will learn to ask yourself questions about your family's health conditions. For example, is it really Attention Deficit Disorder or could it be a mis-diagnosed deficiency of one or more nutrients? Another common question—is your child a slow learner, or could he or she be deficient in protein, in particular the amino acid L-glutamine? Did you know that your husband's bad breath or stinky feet is really body language, as is your teenager's acne? Perhaps the problem your mother or father or even Aunt Susie or Cousin Paul has can be found somewhere within the pages of this book and can be corrected once you recognize the deficiency symptoms. The stories in this book give you examples of common family ailments that can usually be corrected by nutritional means.

Remember, through symptoms, the body is conveying a message that it is at dis-ease, that there is a nutritional deficiency or, in some cases, an overabundance of a particular nutrient. Perhaps you will find your own symptoms between the first and last story of this book and, through improved nutrition, correct the condition. But beware of one danger! Do not postpone medical attention! Self-doctoring can be extremely dangerous. If a condition occurs, you should improve your nutrition, including supplements, and consult a nutritionally oriented physician.

Look at Me, I'm Talking to You! is about those little things I learned to look for in people to help me help them. This book is a how-to manual in true-story form. You can learn to look for the cause of the condition before determining its treatment. An additional note: It might appear to you in reading the stories in this book that I am not an advocate of the medical profession. On the contrary, I wholeheartedly believe in the dedicated people within the medical profession. Unfortunately, most professions have various degrees of talent, and this is true for the medical profession. Some of the people in these stories refer to the inadequacies of their doctor or doctors. This is by no means a reflection on the entire medical profession, just on those few doctors whom my clients had the misfortune of engaging.

This book is a series of real-life incidents that occurred during my years in the vitamin industry. These stories materialized because of the one fundamental practice I consistently engaged in—asking questions. It didn't matter to me if the questions were embarrassing or somewhat personal in nature to my clients, I was on a quest. If I observed something out of the ordinary about a person and I believed that it might be related to a nutritional deficiency, then I asked questions. In retrospect, I'm glad I did. If I hadn't questioned my clients, then the experiences described here and the effect they had on the persons involved would never have occurred. Now, hopefully, you will also benefit.

—Bob

1

Body Language - Cause and Effect

Most retailers, I think, are curious about how others in their field work, compared to their own methods. I know I'm curious about how other vitamin retailers conduct their business. I've discovered many merchandising ideas by visiting other stores, both while on vacation and by going to nearby communities. One time my wife and I were vacationing in Seattle, a most beautiful city. There just happened to be a vitamin store near our hotel and I, of course, found myself looking in the window and then entering the store. A young salesperson greeted me warmly, and I honestly said I was just looking. I didn't tell her that I also worked in a vitamin store—at least not right then.

A few minutes later, a woman entered the store and she, too, was warmly greeted and asked how she could be served.

The woman told the salesperson she was looking for an energy pill—something that would wake her up in the morning and give her energy throughout the day.

I noticed that the woman was dressed in a very heavy coat. Now Seattle does get cold in the winter, but this was early spring and the temperature was probably in the mid-seventies—cool for many and perhaps even chilly for some, but not so cold as to dictate such a thick coat. Of course, I realized there could be many reasons for wearing such warm clothing. Maybe she started out of the house early in the morning when the weather was much colder. Maybe it was the only coat she had. Maybe she gets colder than most people.

I also noticed that she was on the plump side. Was she asking for an energy pill for weight loss? My curiosity got the best of me. I moved to the aisle where the salesperson and this customer were talking. How was the salesperson going to handle this situation? Was she going to ask a series of questions about why her customer had no energy, or was she just going to sell her what she wanted rather than what she might need?

she just looked at me without saying anything, and so I said what I thought she wanted me to say.

"I promise I will be tactful. I promise I will respect all parties concerned."

Her smile told me I had said the right words to put her at ease.

"I guess that none of us has all the answers, not even the best of the best, and as much reading as I do, it never seems to be enough," she said as we moved toward her customer.

"Maureen, telephone." It was another employee calling to my saleslady.

"Get their name and number, and I'll call them back."

"It's the school. Something about your daughter."

"Please excuse me. I must get to the phone. Please, please go on with your ideas. I'll join you as soon as I can." She hurried to the back room of the store. I needed to delay the customer's leaving until my salesperson could get back. I approached the checkout counter where the customer and her saleslady were standing.

"Beautiful day, isn't it?" I asked, looking directly at the customer.

She nodded yes.

"Not too cold and not too warm, just comfortable," I continued.

The young salesperson was probably wondering if I was trying to pick up her customer.

The customer answered, "I think it's rather cold, in fact very cold, at least for me." She turned away after answering.

Yes, I thought, *another symptom determined.*

The young salesperson was totaling up the sale of the energy pill when my saleslady walked up.

"Everything okay, Maureen?" the young saleslady asked.

"Oh yes, Amy just forgot her lunch, so I had to make arrangements with her teacher." Looking at me she continued. "Here you are, sir, these are what you requested," she said as she put the bottles on the counter next to the vitamin A and bioflavonoids I had set down.

Maureen turned her attention to the customer. "Excuse me ma'am, I recognize you as a regular customer, but I've never had the opportunity to introduce myself. My name is Maureen," she said, putting her hand forward.

The customer took Maureen's hand into her own and said, "I am so glad to meet you in person. Your people have helped me so very much, and now I can thank you personally."

"You're welcome," responded Maureen. "In our continuing effort to help you, I would like to introduce you to Bob. He owns a vitamin store in California, and he and I would like to discuss some interesting concepts with you. Again, to better help you. It is okay, isn't it?"

"Why, yes, of course. I just wanted my usual energy pill, but go ahead, let's talk. By the way, my name is Janet."

We shook hands, and I started in. I pushed the vitamin bottles toward Janet. "These are for you. These are the energy pills that your body is asking for." I pointed at the bottle in the young salesperson's hand and said that this energy pill was okay, but not to be taken all of the time.

"May I ask you a couple of questions that you don't have to answer, of course, but if you do, perhaps your answers will determine the real reason you don't have any energy?" I didn't wait for her response, nor did I want either salesperson to interfere at this point.

"Do you bruise easily, do you have a low body temperature, do you have little goose bumps on the back of your arms even when you're not chilled?" I could tell by the look in her eyes that she did indeed have these symptoms. I continued, "Headaches. Do you have both migraine and the usual ones? Do you have respiratory problems such as asthma, and do you have cold hands and feet?" I was overwhelming her with the barrage of questions. Sometimes when I get started, I absolutely cannot stop. Each answer triggers another question.

"Bob, your questions are getting on the personal side. Are they necessary?" asked Maureen.

"Yes, they are. The answers to these questions are crucial in determining Janet's nutritional deficiencies and enabling us to know what to suggest to correct those deficiencies."

I looked at Janet and said, "Please, please excuse me, I do indeed get overzealous about this industry. And, yes, your personal life isn't any of my business, but, in a way, it is. I believe that those of us in this industry really want to help those who are hurting. We help, not by diagnosing or prescribing, but by determining whether a person is deficient in a nutrient that could correct a problem that is causing them to hurt. Let me explain. You asked this salesperson about an energy pill. That prompts many questions in my head. For instance, is your lack of energy from a lack of sleep? If not, then I would ask, 'Do you wake up tired? Why are you wearing such a heavy jacket? Is it because you are constantly cold?' I also noticed that you are squinting, which causes me to look at your fingernails and your hair. The sinus problems and allergies you admitted to prompt questions such as the goose bumps on the back of your arms and constant colds, and, of course, whether you have asthma or even ear infections."

The look in everyone's eyes was of amazement.

I continued. "If your answers to most of my questions were *yes*, I would ask about dizziness when arising from a sitting or lying position." That hit home.

"What about dizziness?" she asked and then continued. "What does it mean if a person gets dizzy after lying down and then getting up?" Instead of answering her question, I asked if it happens to her.

"Yes, and I was so afraid to find out why that I hesitated to go to the doctor, but I finally did. I thought it might be a brain tumor or something."

"And?" I asked.

"No, no brain tumor. He said I was just over-stressed and that my body was responding by causing me to get dizzy." The doctor was partially correct in concluding that stress causes dizziness, but I doubted that the doctor knew why. I didn't tell them my thoughts.

She continued, "He also said my dizziness was because of my allergies. It could have something to do with a possible infection in my ears. But no, no brain tumor or anything like that." She sighed as she completed her sentence, then asked, "What are these bottles all about? How are they going to give me energy? And what about this one—isn't this any good?"

I repeated her question in my mind. No, it really isn't good, at least for her, but I can't give her my honest opinion without creating some doubt in her mind about this vitamin store.

"It's not a question of whether or not this item is any good. The question is, do you want to correct your problem? You can still take the energy pill in addition to these others." I took the energy pill bottle in my hand and added, "This brand is actually very reputable." That wasn't a lie; it's just that I don't necessarily agree with the energy pill concept, but I didn't tell her that. "As for these bottles," I said pointing to the bioflavonoids, "this one corrects what is known as capillary fragility, or more commonly known as bruise marks. You know, those little purple marks that appear when you hit yourself against something."

She nodded yes and then asked, "How did you know I bruise easily? I have on this long-sleeved coat. You couldn't have seen my bruise marks."

"You're right. It was a presumption on my part because you were looking for an energy pill, had on a heavy coat, and..." Instead of answering, I asked, "Do you find yourself gaining weight easily, or do you have difficulty in losing weight?"

"I'm a little fat aren't I? Yes. Yes to all those questions. You're not only good, but tactful as well. Thank you."

"You're welcome," I answered and then continued with my explanation. "These are symptoms of a low thyroid, or hypothyroidism."

"My doctor said my thyroid is okay," she retorted.

"Did you answer *yes* to my question about low body temperature?" I countered.

"Yes. Actually it runs at about 96.5 degrees, but I was told that it is considered low/normal."

I turned to Maureen and asked, "Do you have the book *Hypothyroidism, The Unsuspected Illness* by Dr. Broda Barnes?"

She answered, "Yes, I do. I'll get it." She turned and headed toward the book section.

"While you're there, perhaps you have a book by Adelle Davis..."

I didn't finish my question as I heard my salesperson answer, "I have all of her books. Do you want the one titled *Let's Get Well*?"

"Yes, you're a mind reader," I answered.

"She really is. She knows answers before they're asked. Maureen, I mean. That's my boss. She owns this vitamin store. I think she is psychic," answered the young salesperson.

Maureen came back smiling, having overheard what her salesperson had said. "Thanks, Margie, you're giving away my best-kept secret," she said jokingly. She handed the books to me.

I held up Dr. Barnes's book. "Read this book. It will explain why you have the problems we discussed and many more. This book is truly an eye-opener, especially for those who have been told by their doctor that they don't have a thyroid problem."

Maureen jumped in, "If only we could get more doctors to read this book. I mean, after all, it was written by one of their peers."

I held up the bottle of thyroid substance by Natural Factors. "This could be your primary energizer." I handed the bottle to the customer. I then picked up the bottle of kelp and displayed it in my hand. "Dry hair, brittle fingernails, and eye sensitivity to light. This is, perhaps, why you are squinting."

"Yes, my eyes are sensitive to light. I usually wear my sunglasses even when I'm in a store. I forgot them today, so I squint."

I held up the bottle of vitamin A. "This vitamin, I champion. The medical profession always picks on vitamin A, and yet it is so valuable in maintaining health. For instance, catching cold easily, asthma or bronchial problems, sinusitis, and dry skin are all remedied by vitamin A."

Again, the customer stopped me. "I have all those conditions, but I didn't know that dry skin was a vitamin A deficiency."

"Vitamin A is instrumental in lubricating the skin, and it's especially valuable in lubricating the eyes."

"But isn't vitamin A dangerous? I mean, I heard that it is better to take beta carotene because vitamin A is toxic. Shouldn't she take the beta carotene instead?" asked Margie, the young salesperson.

This time Maureen answered her. "Margie, in this book, the one about hypothyroidism, the doctor explains that people with this affliction cannot easily convert beta carotene to usable vitamin A. It's better that they take natural vitamin A instead." She looked at me, pleased with her answer.

I smiled and nodded yes to her.

"Go on, Bob, I didn't mean to interfere."

I suggested to Maureen that she continue, as she was doing so well. She went on, "Now, how can this vitamin be helpful in providing energy? If a person is deficient in this vitamin, he or she is unable to manufacture the hormone thyroxin in the thyroid gland. So these nutrients—vitamin A, kelp (which contains iodine and is a food for the thyroid), and the thyroid substance itself—help the thyroid gland function more normally. Bioflavonoids are good for..."

"I remember," added Janet. "It's for my awful bruise marks."

I smiled at their increasing enthusiasm.

"What about this one?" Janet asked as she held up the pantothenic acid. "What kind of acid is it?"

"Actually, it is one of the B vitamins, B-5 to be specific, which is customarily indicated for dizziness and the usual headaches. Adelle Davis championed this particular vitamin. It's worth reading her book, too. She refers to pantothenic acid as the 'anti-stress' vitamin."

"So does *Prescription for Nutritional Healing* by Dr. James Balch," chimed in Margie, pleased that she, too, could contribute.

"What about my migraine headaches? Where is the vitamin for that?" asked Janet.

"Janet, I have a theory that migraine headaches are caused by low thyroid. Again, that's only an opinion. I have never read or heard anything to justify my belief, but I have had a lot of success with many of my customers in this regard."

"Bob, can I get your work telephone number? I'd like to continue communicating with you," said Maureen.

We exchanged addresses and telephone numbers, and I thanked them for their tolerance in allowing me to "butt in" with their customer. As I started to leave, I stopped to ask Janet a question. "Janet, I'm writing a book about some of my experiences in nutrition. May I include your story?"

You know her answer.

2

Moist Hands and Blood Sugar

It's fun to ask people questions they don't expect to be asked. My wife, Pat, and I were at a party—a dull party. And although I wanted to go home, Pat asked that we stay. She suggested, "Go play your game of Sherlock Holmes," and then pointed out a comfortable-looking chair next to the refreshments. I heeded her advice, filled my glass with punch and my hand with some unhealthy goodies, and sat in the inviting chair.

When at a party I usually promise my wife that I will forget my job unless, of course, there is a situation where a deficiency is so apparent that I have to say something to the person afflicted.

This time I saw a male guest, with drink in hand, talking to two young ladies. His hand trembled as he held his glass, a clue to a possible blood sugar problem or a symptom of some illness. I also noticed his fingernails. They had several very prominent white spots on them. Oh, I know, your mom, as did mine, said that this was caused by telling lies. Actually, it's a deficiency of the mineral zinc.

I recall my years as an adolescent, when most of the teenage boys had those white spots on their fingernails. Now, years later, I realize that they were the same ones who usually had the worst cases of acne. Acne is also associated with a deficiency of zinc, which helps the skin to heal. However, the male guest I was watching at the party was in his late fifties or early sixties. Obviously, he would not be a candidate for adolescent acne, but he could have a prostate problem. If he were at my store, I would ask him several additional questions relating to a deficiency of zinc, but I was at a party and I did promise Pat not to be an active Sherlock Holmes. I kept quiet, which is difficult for me to do when someone's health could be in jeopardy. I looked away from him and allowed my eyes to wander over the rest of the guests.

Yes, I did see other symptoms. The gal with slumped shoulders was probably lacking minerals. And the older woman with crippling arthritis—was her doctor treating her nutritionally as well as with drugs? Of course, one can always observe the bags or dark circles under someone's eyes, and other deficiency symptoms such as dry hair, which could, of course, be caused by hair spray, but then again it could also be a symptom of thyroid dysfunction.

"Bob?"

I looked up at the sound of my name.

"Bob, hi, how are you?" A tall blonde-haired woman with a lovely smile greeted me. She extended her hand to me, which I promptly took. It was neither cold nor moist.

"Bob, I'm so glad you're here. I want you to meet a dear friend of mine," she said with a wink and then whispered, "I hope more than a dear friend." I got up from my most comfortable chair to meet the apparent new man in her life.

"John," she said to the man holding the glass. "I'm sorry, ladies, for interrupting, but I want John to meet Bob. They have so much in common."

The two ladies smiled their approval and stepped back as Katie introduced me to John, the guy with the white spots on his nails. She also introduced me to the two ladies. We exchanged our hello's and glad-to-meet-you's, and then they excused themselves and turned away.

"John, this is Bob Weiss. He and his wife, Pat, are the ones who own Bob Cannon's Vitamin Stores. They and their staff have helped me countless times."

John put his drink in his left hand in order for us to exchange handshakes. He had a good grip, which is healthy, but I could not help but notice that his hand was very moist. Yes, it could have been from the cold glass, but it did cause me to wonder if his hands were always moist. I also wondered if he was bothered with headaches. Did he have a temper? As we began conversing, I looked at his eyes for signs of allergies.

It was then that Katie dropped her empty hors d'oeuvre plate. John bent down to pick it up, and he did not immediately stand back up, but got up very slowly. I couldn't help myself.

"Bad back?" I asked.

"No, I just like getting up slowly. I don't want to hurt my back so I take it a little slower than I used to."

Hmmm, not the answer I expected. "Good reasoning," I said. "More people at our age should be as cautious as you." I pushed for the answer I was expecting. "Although I never had a bad back, I used to have to get up slowly; otherwise, I would get a little woozy."

"You mean dizzy, like the room was spinning around?" asked Katie.

I answered, "Yes."

"John, you complained to me just the other day that you sometimes get dizzy when you get up too fast."

Bingo. I was right, but it was unfortunate for John, having this problem. Or was it? Now he knows someone who might be able to help him. I don't think John appreciated what Katie revealed; he glared at her. She blushed and whispered, "I'm sorry." He patted her hand and took it in his and smiled at her. I wondered if Katie noticed his moist hands, or was she too much in like or love to notice?

The three of us talked for a short while, mostly about nutrition. Then I asked John what he did for a living. He told me that he was a retired schoolteacher. He had taught science and coached sports. At this point, the hostess called to Katie. As she departed, she said, "John, talk to Bob. He's a good guy." With that, she turned away and walked across the room.

"No, I'm not, John," I said.

"Not what?" he asked.

He either didn't hear what Katie had said or his thoughts were elsewhere.

"Katie said that I'm a good guy, and I'm not."

"Oh, I'm sure you are; otherwise, Katie wouldn't have said so. What makes you say that you're not?" he asked.

"I get too nosey at times," I answered.

"In what way? I mean, nosey about what?"

This opened the door for me. Now I could ask him about things I had suspected. John told me he was a recovering alcoholic. That would explain the moist hands, the dizziness on arising, and the dark circles under his eyes. His pancreas, adrenal glands, and maybe even his kidneys could be affected.

"John, have you experienced any problems with your prostate gland?"

He answered that he had.

The following Monday both John and Katie came into my store to complete a Body Language Questionnaire. Based on his answers, I could tell his body required zinc, pantothenic acid, all of the B vitamins, E, C and a multiple mineral complex. He decided to purchase them all, as well as Cheramino, a liquid protein supplement I suggested. Within a week his headaches were, as he said, 90 percent better. His dizziness was almost completely gone, and he had an unexpected increase in energy—sustained energy, as he called it.

He also admitted that he had not had a temper tantrum. "I don't seem to have road rage anymore, or at least it's lessening. Is it my imagination or am I taking something for this problem as well?"

"John, you've improved your diet considerably, especially by including the Cheramino with breakfast and between lunch and dinner. You're getting the protein your body has been craving. Yes, this could lessen your temper by leveling your blood sugar content."

John was certainly on the road to recovery and should continue in that direction as long as he maintained a sensible eating program.

Katie and John never did get married. A couple of months after he visited my store, John was in an auto accident requiring that he take several prescription drugs for the intense pain. Unfortunately, this caused him to start drinking once again. Eventually he moved from the area. Katie said that John was too embarrassed to be seen by his friends in his drunken condition, so he moved to Arizona to, as he put it, "dry out again." Katie never heard from him and eventually moved back to Atlanta.

3

ALCOHOLISM

"Can you help me?" is a question I've been asked many times throughout my career. A young man in his early twenties came into my store one afternoon and asked me that question. He reeked of beer and cigarette smoke—the nauseating stench eventually filled the store. His clothes were disheveled and his hair was uncombed. His wanting some help meant he was about to ask for some money or other handout.

"Can you help me?" he asked, once again.

"Maybe. What kind of help are you in need of?" I asked. I wasn't ready for the answer he was about to give.

"I just came from that dungeon next door, and I don't want to be one of them. Can you help me?" he pleaded.

The "dark dungeon next door" was how he described a local beer bar two-doors from my store. His not wanting to be "one of them" caught me off guard. My heart was starting to open up to this stranger, but I also knew I had to be wary. I looked into his dark, gray, bloodshot eyes. Too much beer, I assumed. But he had asked for help, so I decided to see the extent of the help he wanted. I started by introducing myself and putting forth my hand. I needed to touch his to determine if my suspicions were correct.

"My name is Bob. What's yours?"

"Jason," he said as he put his hand in mine.

As I expected, his hand was moist. Moist hands indicate trouble with the pancreas and/or the adrenal glands.

"Jason, are there any blood sugar problems in your family? Do your parents or grandparents on either side have hypoglycemia, diabetes, or alcoholism?"

"Yes. Both my mom and dad are alcoholics. So is my older brother. Am I going to end up like them?"

"Jason, there are several things that could help you with your problem. We have to determine if you are deficient in each of them before you spend any money."

"How much is it going to cost?"

"Again, that depends on your needs and how quickly you wish to get help."

He reached into his pocket and pulled out a bundle of money. The bills were in total disarray. Bent, crumpled, twisted, they had the stench of alcohol and cigarette smoke. One by one he straightened them out, placing them on the counter.

"I have eleven dollars and some change. That's all I've got. But I do get paid on Friday. I can come back on Friday and finish up what I need."

Eleven dollars to correct a problem. There was only one product that would give him immediate, but not long-lasting, help. I walked over to the protein section and took a bottle of Cheramino, a liquid predigested protein.

"Here, Jason." I handed him the bottle.

"What do I do with it?"

"If you have a tablespoon handy, take a spoonful four times a day. If not, take a swig right from the bottle, again four times a day. If you feel as if you really need a drink, take another tablespoon full or another swig."

"And then what?" he asked.

"If you're satisfied with the results, and that means you won't want a beer, you'll be back on Friday to buy some more. I discounted the price on this bottle; however, I'll have to charge you full price for the next bottle."

"What does it taste like?"

"Jason, it tastes like cherry-flavored motor oil. You might not like how it tastes, but your body's desire for protein will offset that."

Jason came back on Saturday. He had not had a beer or any alcohol since he started the liquid protein. During the next few weeks, he added several other supplements, including a multivitamin, magnesium, ginseng, chromium, and pantothenic acid. Over the next several months Jason would report on his progress, and he was progressing. And then I didn't see him for three weeks. I knew he wasn't on vacation as that wouldn't be for three months. I could only wonder what had happened to him. A customer who was also a team leader and counselor at Alcohol Anonymous told me that supplements alone wouldn't help Jason. He needed counseling in addition to his vitamin regimen; otherwise, he was doomed for failure.

Another week passed before Jason returned to my store. He was dressed in a dark blue suit, wore a snazzy tie, and his shoes were shined to the rim. He certainly didn't look as if he had fallen off the wagon and back into drinking. This was not the same Jason who had come in to the store eight months ago.

"Bob, I've been working in Colorado this past month; that's why you haven't seen me. My job sent me there to see if I could handle the weather. Bob, I've received a promotion, which means I'll be moving to Colorado. I don't know how to ever thank you for giving me the help and support I needed way back when. I haven't had a drink of any kind for eight months, and I absolutely do not have any desire for one."

About a year later, Jason wrote to me saying he was still clean, the job was going well, and he was engaged to be married.

It's very gratifying to help someone who is willing to help himself.

4

Manic-Depression/Bipolar Disorder

"Her kids are manic-depressive and also bipolar, the same as my daughter Tanya. She, too, had both of those illnesses." Jill, my new neighbor, was referring to another of our neighbors, who lived across the street from us. Actually, it was my wife and I who were the new neighbors. We had just moved into the city two months earlier.

"Poor Lila. She has three children to cope with."

"Jill, I thought that manic-depression and bipolar were the same, except that bipolar was the medical term."

"No, they're different," Jill responded. I didn't challenge her answer.

"Let me ask you a few questions about your daughter, if you don't mind."

"It's okay."

"Jill, I'm not being nosey. I do nutritional counseling; consequently, I have a tendency to ask a lot of questions."

"Go ahead, Bob, get nosey. Ask what you want."

"Does your daughter have mood swings?"

"Yes."

"Are the palms of her hands always moist?"

"Yes."

"Does she suffer from headaches on a daily basis?"

"Yes."

"Does she complain of dizziness upon rising? Does she have allergies? Does she have vague fears? Does she ache all over?"

"Yes, yes, yes."

"Jill, if I'm asking too fast, tell me to slow down."

"No. You're doing fine."

"Does she have a poor appetite and, when she does eat, does she prefer sugar foods such as bread, pasta..."

"And candy and soft drinks and bread. She would even eat catsup sandwiches. Just catsup and bread." she answered.

After asking Jill all of these questions and getting all *yes* answers, I was somewhat surprised that my questions hadn't aroused her curiosity. I continued.

"Jill, has your daughter ever tried suicide?" I knew that I was really getting personal, and I hoped Jill wouldn't be too upset.

"Oh, Bob, didn't you know? My daughter died two years ago. She locked herself in her bathroom and slashed her wrists while in the bathtub. Unfortunately, she was one of the small percentage of those afflicted with this illness who take their own lives."

I was taken aback. Then I wondered why she allowed me to ask all of those questions in the present tense, but I didn't pursue this. After extending my apologies and condolences, I decided to say nothing more, as there wasn't anything I could do. We stood quietly for a short while, and then Jill broke the silence.

"My Tanya was adopted. I later found out that both her real mother and father were also manic-depressive. The doctor said that it could be an inherited trait."

"Jill, were they also alcoholics or drug addicts?" Because Jill re-opened the conversation, I felt I could ask this question.

"I don't know about drugs, but, yes, they were alcoholics. I don't know about Lila's three children. I know that they, too, are adopted, but I don't believe Lila has their medical history."

"Do you know how Lila would answer the questions I just asked you?"

"You would get the same answers. We've already compared notes."

"Jill, has anyone ever asked you those same questions before, including the doctor?"

"No, not exactly. He did ask if Tanya was moody. And she was."

"All of the questions I asked you were related to deficiencies of different nutrients. If Lila were to answer *yes* to them, perhaps we, or I, could give her some diet ideas."

"Bob, you don't understand. My Tanya and Lila's children are mentally ill. There isn't any vitamin that can help them."

"Maybe not. But what if those symptoms, at least, could be corrected or lessened by taking supplements? Wouldn't that be of some benefit?"

"Bob, it's a mental disease, not a nutritional deficiency," she answered most adamantly.

Over the next couple of weeks I discovered that Lila, too, was fully convinced that nutrition did not play a part in her children's problem. She also concluded that it was a mental condition only, and that no amount of vitamins could help them. In my opinion, both of these women had been brainwashed. If it were my children, I would at the very least be curious enough to try anything, as long as it didn't interfere with their medication.

In asking Jill those questions, I had made a preliminary conclusion that Tanya had been deficient in protein, the B vitamins, especially pantothenic acid, and vitamin C. I also suspected that her adrenal glands, as well as her pancreas, were in need of some nutritional help. I would have also suggested that she consider the amino acids taurine and L-tyrosine. I also believe that the essential fatty acids play an extremely important role as well. One might ask, "An oil for the brain?" Oil is a fat, and the brain is primarily made up of fat. For Tanya, I was too late. For Lila's three children, she was too closed-minded to consider my suggestions.

5

Skin - Sensitivity to Touch

"Ouch. Stop it, Jim, that hurts."

"Oh, you're just too sensitive."

"I don't care what you think, it hurts, and it's embarrassing."

Jim, who was getting bored with shopping, patted his wife on the buttocks, suggested that she hurry, and said, "We have a long ride ahead of us."

Jim and Lois lived a distance from my store, but they made the trip at least once a month.

"Lois," I asked, "are you really that sensitive? Jim didn't seem to hit you all that hard; it appeared to be more of a pat."

"Oh, Bob, it stings. I could feel it throughout my entire body."

"Are you also sensitive to bug bites, including mosquitoes and fleas?"

"Terribly. I can't go anywhere after dark without wearing a long-sleeved shirt and something to cover my neck. And even with all that covering, they still attack my hands and face."

"Are you being treated for any heart conditions?"

"No, but, according to the doctor, I do have an erratic heartbeat. It sometimes speeds up and then it slows down, and then it returns to normal. He did some tests, which were negative; I mean my heart was okay. He suggested we just keep an eye on it and see if it gets any worse."

"Are you taking your multiple vitamin?"

"No," she answered somewhat sheepishly. "I can't swallow those horse pills; I feel as if I'm going to choke."

"Do you have any other fears, I mean, something that's not really explainable?"

"Jim thinks I'm weird. I have strange fears—no, vague fears—about everything. I didn't mention them to the doctor because I don't want to take any prescription drugs."

"Lois, would you prefer taking your multivitamin as powder in a drink? Or a capsule that you can separate and add to some juice?"

"I guess the capsule. Yes, I can add it to juice and Jim can swallow his. I just can't swallow pills."

I walked over to the vitamin B section of the store and returned with a bottle of vitamin B-1 in my hand.

"Lois, this is a tablet about the size of a baby aspirin. Do you believe you would have trouble swallowing a pill this small?"

"Probably."

"You can break or crush this little pill and add that to your juice as well. You take your multivitamin with either breakfast or lunch and one of these pills at dinnertime. You are very deficient in vitamin B-1. I also noticed just now that your tongue is very red—too red—which indicates still other deficiencies."

"Can I start these after next week? Jim and I are going camping up at the High Sierras for a week."

"Yes, you can, unless you don't want to be bothered by mosquitoes while you're camping."

"What do you mean?"

"Vitamin B-1 has helped many of my customers either lessen the effects of bug bites or eliminate them completely. As for your skin sensitivity and irregular heartbeat, those conditions might take a little longer."

Lois started taking her vitamins that evening and continued her regimen for the next month. That's when the couple returned to my store. After our mutual greetings, Lois told Jim to sit down while she told her success stories. No bug bites, and the heart palpitations had almost completely stopped. "My doctor was pleased about that."

"What about your strange fears and your skin sensitivity—any progress in those areas?"

"Bob, I'm less fearful of everything, but I need to ask you a favor about the skin sensitivity. Please don't tell Jim what I'm about to say. I absolutely don't have that 'all-over-hurt' feeling anymore. But please, please don't tell Jim. I'm letting him believe that it still stings when he slaps my behind, but it doesn't. I just don't want him doing it anymore."

6

EYES...AND DARK CIRCLES

Although Linda was discussing her nutritional problems with some of my sales staff, I could not help but notice the dark circles under her eyes. Allergies, kidney problems, or weak adrenal glands were my first thoughts. Unfortunately, my sales staff was so bewildered by her other crises that they paid no attention to her eyes. Finally, I was invited into the conversation for my opinion.

Linda was allergic to soy, wheat, soft cheeses, whey, yogurt, and bread and yet could eat ice cream and drink milk. She had been to many medical doctors and several of our competitors, but to no avail. No one had an answer for her. Yes, she was on medication for her problem, but its success had been minimal. As I walked toward Linda, I noticed her head was tilted to one side. We were introduced, and she began telling me her story. As she talked, I looked for obvious deficiencies. The most noticeable was revealed by her teeth. She had poor teeth displacement, my first clue suggesting a calcium deficiency. Her hair seemed dry, and as she talked her head continued tilting from one side to the other. Another clue, this one indicating weak adrenal glands, which would explain the dark circles under her eyes.

I asked, "Do you have airborne allergies as well?" I knew the answer would be *yes,* and it was.

"Do you have headaches?" Again I knew the answer would be *yes*. She added that her headaches had been diagnosed as migraines.

"Are you on medication for the migraines?"

"Yes," she answered and then added, "but to no avail."

"Do have episodes of itchy skin?"

Another *yes* and then she said, "Especially when I have my breakouts from my eating allergies. Over the weekend I had a taste for cheese, and this is the result." She showed me several spots on her arms, upper legs, and tummy. "This really itches me."

"May I touch your hand?" I asked.

With a smile she answered yes by extending her hand and placing it into mine.

One of my staff said, "Don't worry, Linda, Bob always touches people's hands. It's for a reason."

Her hands were definitely cold, too cold for weather that was currently in the high 90s.

"Well?" she asked.

"Do you also have cold feet?"

"My hands aren't cold. Are my hands cold?" she asked as she extended her hand to one of my sales staff. My employee took Linda's hand into hers and then put the back of Linda's own hand up to Linda's face.

"Oh, they are a little chilly," said Linda. "What does that mean? I mean, my mom has cold hands. I guess it runs in the family."

I answered her by asking if she recently had some ice cream or drank some milk.

She answered no, she hadn't had anything to eat since early that morning. It was now two in the afternoon. Linda apparently had not eaten in six or more hours and yet her tongue was very coated.

"Aren't you a little hungry?" I asked. She answered yes, but added that she was trying to maintain her weight. I guessed Linda at being about a size 4 and later learned she was a size 2. I could only guess that she was starving herself to maintain her slim figure.

"Well, Mr. Bob, what's your opinion?" she asked.

I suggested she take home one of our nutritional profiles so we could provide a more in-depth answer for her.

"I leave in two days for San Francisco. What can you tell me now?"

"Are you moving from our area?"

"No, my job takes me across the country, and this week it happens to be in San Francisco. I'll be back next week. Please, tell me something," she pleaded.

"Linda, I suspect low thyroid."

"Wow, that's news to me. How did you determine that?"

"There were several indications, but we'll know more after you do the profile questionnaire and this underarm test." I handed her an instruction sheet that my employee had retrieved when Linda confirmed her cold hands.

She quickly read it and said that we'll all have to wait for the results. "At least three more weeks," she added with a grin. (The underarm thyroid test is best done on the second, third, and fourth day of a woman's menstrual cycle. Linda was obviously three weeks away from that time.)

I continued, "These are the symptoms of a deficiency of pantothenic acid." I handed her a sheet of paper that listed in great detail the many symptoms of a deficiency of this important B vitamin. As Linda started to read the list, I continued talking to her.

"I also suspect that you are deficient in hydrochloric acid and/or enzymes. These supplements assist in the digestion of food. In my opinion, if a person has adequate stomach acid, allergies to food are almost impossible."

"That's quite a statement, and to you it seems logical, but I don't understand. How—I mean—what are the reasons for your opinions? At the doctor's office they take blood tests, check my blood pressure, my temperature, and give me their opinion based on the results of the testing. You just ask me questions, touch my hands, look at my tongue, and already have opinions. I don't understand how you can reach these conclusions so quickly."

"When they took your temperature, was it lower than normal?"

"Yes. They said it was on the low side. They also said my blood pressure was on the low side as well, but that everything was okay in that regard."

"Did they advise you that you might have a low thyroid condition?"

"No, of course not, and yet you tell me that I do just by asking me questions."

"Linda, some of the deficiency symptoms of low thyroid include cold hands and feet. You also said you had difficulty maintaining your weight, you have migraine headaches, and both your body temperature and blood pressure are on the low side. Accumulatively, this indicates low thyroid. As for the other conclusions, it started with the dark circles under your eyes, your teeth, your tongue, your many allergies, including food and airborne, and the tilting of your head from side to side. I also suspect you have painful menstrual cramping, difficulty falling asleep, or leg cramps. Maybe all three."

"I do. Have all three symptoms, I mean."

"Most of these items are mentioned on the nutritional profile. I was just asking you the questions, but now you can take this questionnaire with you to San Francisco and bring the results back to us when you get home."

"First," she said, "I'm going to buy the three things you mentioned—pantothenic acid, enzymes, and hydrochloric acid. I need help, and although I'm not a hundred percent positive about your findings, it does make sense. At least, I think so."

Linda bought these items, and we all wished her well. I could hardly wait for her return to hear the results.

Linda returned from her trip to San Francisco and came into my store with the completed profile in hand. I read what she had answered and was satisfied that what she had bought two weeks earlier was indeed indicated.

"What else do I need?" she asked.

"Before I answer your question, please tell me, how are you feeling since taking the pantothenic acid, hydrochloric acid, and the enzymes? And not necessarily in that order."

"Bob, I can't begin to tell you how much better I feel. I've been taking the pantothenic acid whenever I feel a headache coming on. It really helps; in fact, my headaches are getting less severe and less frequent. Is my head tilting anymore?" she asked with a chuckle. "I told my sister about what I'm taking and how you look at people to determine what vitamin they're deficient in. She sort of scoffed at it. She also told me not to take the hydrochloric acid because of my condition."

"What condition is that? Is it something we have discussed?"

"I get a lot of bladder infections and, no, I hadn't told you. Anyway, my sister—oh, by the way, she is a surgeon at one of L.A.'s leading hospitals—she said that the hydrochloric acid, because of being an acid, would make my condition worse. But the enzymes seem to be working just fine. What do you suggest?"

"I suggest you follow your doctor's advice. Linda, let's talk about your being too acidic. Are you familiar with the term *pH*?"

"Yes, that's the acid/alkaline balance your body is in."

"Did you know that minerals play the primary role in determining your pH balance?"

"Yes, at least I think I knew that."

"Did you also know that if a person is deficient in hydrochloric acid he or she is unable to assimilate most minerals? Your answers on the questionnaire regarding hydrochloric acid indicates that you are very deficient, thus, you have a difficult time assimilating minerals. This could lead to an improper pH balance and affect calcium absorption, which ultimately leads to menstrual cramping, leg cramps, difficulty sleeping, and poor teeth displacement. You indicated having all of these symptoms. Linda, do you remember our first meeting and you asked how I knew about your being deficient in Hcl? Your teeth and your tongue tipped me off, and now your profile has established the extent of that deficiency."

"Bob, again I ask, should I take the hydrochloric acid based on what you just told me?"

"No. Let's listen to the doctor. Besides, the enzymes, based on what you've told me, seem to be doing just fine. Linda, now the big question. Have you considered trying any of the foods that you have been allergic to since taking these three supplements?"

"Yes, Bob, I have. I am beginning to have so much confidence in what we're doing. This is the first time I have had any relief, either from my headaches or my eating problems. I'm going away again next week on another business trip and I don't want to experiment at that time. When I get back we'll talk about it."

Early one afternoon three weeks later, a smiling Linda entered the store. She radiated.

"It works! It works!" she almost yelled out. "I tried several of my most allergic foods and it works—the enzymes, I mean. First I tried some yogurt. Just half a teaspoon at first because I guess I was a little scared. It went down fine and I didn't get the usual weird feeling, so I tried to eat a spoonful. Still no weird feeling, so I ate the whole carton. Absolutely no reaction, even hours later. I did take two enzymes before my first bite and then two more after I ate the whole carton. I felt good about it, so later that evening I went for the gusto—pizza with lots of cheese. That's when I got worried. Even though I took four enzymes, I still had a funny feeling about it so I took two hydrochloric acid pills and nothing happened. No rash, no itching, no anything. The next day I took it a little easy and ate my usual safe foods. I didn't want to overburden my body. But the following day I experimented again, and once again the enzymes and hydrochloric acid worked. I called my sister, you know, the surgeon, and told her about my results. She, well, she is a doctor so she's a little leery about the whole thing, but I think that when she and I have lunch together she'll see for herself how I'm doing. And I am doing fine, thanks to you."

7

Thyroid - Cold Hands and Feet

Even though I've retired from my retail store, I will never, never retire from looking at people in terms of their nutritional needs.

One evening I took a break from writing and suggested to my wife that we go out for dinner at a new restaurant.

About the time we were served our meal, a young family was seated next to us. As they settled in their seats and picked up their menus, the daughter, who was about twelve years old, said to her mother, "Mom, I'm cold."

Her mother replied, "It is rather chilly in here. Dad will get your sweater from the car."

"Why didn't you think of that before we came in here? You're always cold—both you and your mom," the father complained.

"Honey, if you're cold, I'll get you your sweater from the car," the mother said.

"That's okay. I'll suffer."

They continued reading the menu, and when the waitress reappeared they placed their order.

"They're both slightly overweight," I whispered to my wife.

She looked up at me as if to say, "Oh no, Bob, we're having a wonderful dinner. Don't get involved." But she didn't say anything, so I continued.

"They could both have a low thyroid condition. The daughter inherited the problem from her mom, who probably inherited it from one or both of her parents."

"Bob, it's no use telling you it isn't any of our business, but I guess that's you. It'll always be your business. Always trying to end someone's misery nutritionally. Can't you at least wait until we're finished with our meal?"

I promised I would.

Just as the family was being served their dinner, the mother got up and said she was going to the car to get her daughter's sweater.

"But Mom, it's okay, I'm not that cold."

The father called out, "Honey, I'll get it." But that was of no avail; the mother was determined to be the one to get the sweater.

We were just completing our dinner when the mother returned. She had two sweaters, one for her daughter and the second she was now wearing.

As our waitress was handing us our check, she noticed that they had put on their sweaters and asked, "Are you cold? I can ask the manager to check the temperature in here. It seems okay, but then again, I have been bustling around, so I don't notice if it does get cold."

"No, we're just fine. Anyway—oh, I'm always cold."

That was my clue. Pat smiled at me and said that she would wait for me at the front of the restaurant. I whispered to her, "Thank you, my love."

I directed my first question at the mother, "And do you also have cold feet?"

"Do you know my wife?" asked the father.

At first I thought he was challenging me for asking the question, but he continued. "She has the coldest feet in the world. How did you know?" he asked laughing.

The mother turned to me and nodded yes and continued, "I always have cold feet and cold hands, especially the fingertips. I guess that I just have poor circulation."

I continued, "—and you bruise easily." It was a statement rather than a question.

The mother looked at me surprised. I couldn't tell if she wondered who this guy was asking her these questions or how did he know that she had all these symptoms. Maybe both.

Again she nodded yes and affirmed it orally, then asked the usual question, "How did you know?"

"An educated guess. Do you also have heart palpitation?"

"I do," chimed in the daughter. "Mom, I told you about my heart, it acts as if it's fluttering or something." The daughter then looked in my direction. "And I have cold hands and cold feet too." she exclaimed.

"Like mother, like daughter," the father commented.

Somewhat annoyed at her husband, the mother gave him a look. "Yes, I do, too, but the doctor said it was just stress. Actually I've been treated for my heart condition for the past three years but it never gets better, or worse for that matter. It's just there, and now I guess I should be concerned about my daughter, Amy. She probably has what I have."

They still hadn't asked who I was or why I was asking these questions. I directed several more questions to both mother and daughter—questions related to a low thyroid condition. Almost in unison, they answered yes to each question I asked.

"Mom, have you ever had your thyroid gland checked by your doctor?" I asked, referring to the mother as "Mom."

She answered that, according to her doctor, there was no reason to go to the expense of testing her thyroid. "The doctor told me it was the heart we should be concerned with."

"Did your parents, either your mother or father, have a thyroid condition?"

She answered that her mother did; it was discovered when she tried dieting. "Maybe that's why I can't lose weight. Do you think it's my thyroid?"

I suggested she visit one of our retail outlets and request a Body Language Questionnaire. I also told her that, although the questionnaire is not designed to diagnose, it does give certain indications that should be pursued further by a medical doctor.

This is why I get involved with people in whom I see a symptom of a deficiency. This young woman had been treated for three years for a heart condition that probably didn't exist. Three years of treating a symptom rather than the cause, which was, based on her many *yes* answers to my questions, probably her thyroid gland. Hopefully, for the sake of the mother and her daughter as well, the doctor will accept the fact that there is a correlation between the heart and the thyroid gland.

I also asked the two ladies questions relating to vitamin A and kelp. (These supplements and their association with low thyroid are discussed in other stories of this book.)

Heart palpitations are not always caused by hypothyroidism, of course, but it should be considered as a possible culprit.

8

Hyperthyroidism

Mary couldn't sit, or even stand still. She talked as she walked, and she walked all around the store as she talked! Having a conversation with her was difficult. Her friend Larry had suggested she see me because of her obvious nervous condition.

"I'm tired of taking nerve pills." she said. "They're making me even more jumpy."

"But look at all of the energy you're burning," I teased. "That's what's keeping you so tiny around the waist."

Mary was in her early fifties, about five-feet-two, and weighed maybe 100 pounds. She was a little too thin for her frame. "Wiry" is how Larry described her. He also said she had a good appetite, but just couldn't gain any weight.

In only a few short minutes Mary convinced me that there were deficiencies associated with her thyroid gland. When Larry first introduced us, I shook Mary's hand; it was unusually warm. She had a flushed look about her, even though there was a slight chill in the room. There was also a slight protrusion of her eyeballs.

She was more than just nervous, she was hyperactive and talked rapidly. She said she had a good appetite but could not gain weight. Larry had also told me that she suffered from a fast heartbeat. These were all symptoms of a fast-acting, perhaps even toxic, thyroid gland.

"Mary," I asked, "have you ever had your thyroid gland checked?"

"Yes. They said it was okay."

"They?" I asked.

"Yes. I've been to three doctors. I was concerned about being so thin, so I went to see my doctor. He sent me to his partner who specializes in weight problems. He put me on a program whereby I actually lost about seven pounds. But I wanted to gain weight, so I stopped seeing him. The next one...well, he's also treating me for my nervous condition."

"Did all three of these doctors check you for a thyroid condition?" I repeated my question.

"My own doctor did, but he said it was fine. I guess he told the others that it was okay because they never checked it."

"Do you have trouble sleeping?" I asked.

"Yes, I suffer from insomnia."

"Mary, it's time for you to go shopping," I said.

"Larry, I like this guy. He knows how to get to a woman's heart."

"No, not that kind of shopping. You need to shop for a doctor—one that's familiar with the thyroid gland, in particular, hyperthyroidism."

"Can't you help me with that?"

"There are several supplements that will help, but it's better that you get a qualified doctor's opinion first."

"Can't I be taking some of these pills until I find a doctor? I really need some help."

"Only if you promise to find that doctor, and soon."

"Bob," said Larry, "I promise you that we'll start, once we get back into our area and that will be in about an hour. In fact, I know of one doctor a friend of mine goes to. He specializes in what they call hormone therapy. Does he sound like the right doctor?"

"I would suggest you at least start with him. Make sure he suggests Mary's thyroid gland be checked. If he determines what I suspect, perhaps he and I can work in tandem as far as supplementation and diet are concerned."

How fortunate it was for Mary that this doctor turned out to be open-minded. Yes, he determined through thorough testing that Mary had hyperthyroidism. He also conferred with me about her diet, although what he suggested was more than adequate. He did tell Mary to take a B-complex plus vitamins E and C and the minerals calcium and magnesium. The amount of iodine he prescribed could only be obtained through the pharmacy.

Mary called me a week later and told me of her progress. She and Larry both called several months later to say goodbye. They were moving to Alaska. How was she doing? She said that her life had been changed and that she was a normal human being again. She had also gained about ten pounds and was no longer on medication for nerves.

9

Depression and Suicide

"Good morning and Happy Tuesday," I greeted my first customer of the day as she entered our store.

"And a good morning to you, too. And, I guess, Happy Tuesday as well."

"What do you mean 'I guess'? Isn't it a happy Tuesday?"

"It's a beautiful Tuesday. It's just, well, I have never heard that expression before. Do you always greet someone with 'Happy Tuesday'?

"Only on Tuesdays," I answered.

"Why only on Tuesdays?"

I smiled.

"Oh, now I get it. Tomorrow it'll be Happy Wednesday and Thursday it'll be... That's a good greeting. Yes, it is a beautiful Tuesday and thanks for making me really aware of it. But then again I guess I should have expected something like that, based on what my friends have said about you and this store."

"Dare I ask?"

"You're people who care, that's what they say. People who care."

She was a typical first-time customer in that she came in because of a referral. That's how my wife, Pat, and I acquired most of our new customers. It was a lot less costly than paying for advertising.

"Could I have one of those, what do you call them, tests? Just what are they?"

"It is not a test but a profile of your deficiencies based on how you answer the questions."

"Can I have two of them? Maybe I can get my husband to do one as well."

"Is there anything in particular you are trying to correct?"

"Yes, of course. Doesn't everyone have problems?"

Instead of answering her question, I showed her how to complete the Body Language Questionnaire.

It was then that another customer entered the store. She was young, possibly in her late teens, maybe very early twenties, but she walked as if she were considerably older, as if she were carrying a heavy burden on her slumping shoulders. I didn't realize that this would be one of the most touching experiences I would ever have.

I greeted her and then asked what she was looking for so that I could point her in the proper direction. She said she was looking for energy pills.

"They're halfway down the aisle, left-hand side, and on the top two shelves."

She smiled, almost whispered a "Thank you," and moved in the direction I had suggested.

The first customer then commented to me, "Such a pretty little thing. But she looks so sad."

I concurred and continued instructing her on the questionnaire and answering her questions; but I couldn't help glancing at the young girl, who seemed to be staring into space rather than at the bottles on the shelf. I was about to ask her if she had found what she was looking for when she turned and started toward the checkout counter. I thought she was going to ask me a question, but she only said, "Thank you," and continued toward the door. I hurriedly asked, "Didn't you find what you were looking for?"

"No. You don't have the kind I use," she answered curtly.

"Yes, I do, it's, ah, it's in the back room," I lied. "I'll get it for you shortly."

She turned and looked at me. There was a quizzical look on her face and before she could say anything I quickly asked her another question.

"Did you want a case or just a couple of bottles?"

"Oh no, I only want one bottle." She still had that quizzical look on her face but accepted my answer and went back to the energy section.

I didn't want her to leave, and yet I didn't want my other first time customer to leave either.

"Go ahead and help her, Bob. She looks as if she could use some help. Anyway, I'll see you again tomorrow with the completed body profiles." She placed the profiles in her purse and started for the exit, stopped, turned to look at me, and then whispered, "She never mentioned what brand she wanted, did she? At least I didn't hear her if she did. Tell me what happens with that little girl."

I said I would, thanked her again, and waved goodbye as she left the store. I started toward the young girl and began reading her body language. I could see from the way she stood why she wanted to buy energy pills, but it was an item I didn't want to sell her.

The slumping of her shoulders gave me my first clue that she was probably deficient in minerals. To confirm this I would have to ask her if she had difficulty sleeping, suffered from leg cramps, or if she had menstrual cramping. Due to her age, the question would be more difficult, but if she did suffer from this problem it would be nice to have it corrected. As I got nearer to her she turned and looked at me and, just as quickly, turned away. I asked myself if she would be too embarrassed to discuss her situation.

Again she turned toward me. Her sorrowful eyes prompted my first question. "How bad is your headache?" I asked in a positive tone, as I already knew what the answer would be.

"Oh, it's bad, but sometimes they're really bad." Once again she turned away from me.

"Your dizziness, just how bad does that get?"

She turned toward me and with a look of astonishment asked, "How did you know I get dizzy? How did you know I have a headache?"

I looked at her eyes. At her young age they should have been a clear blue color just like the sky, but instead they had tinges of gray. Before I could answer, she continued. "Are you psychic or something? How did you know?"

Instead of answering her questions, I continued asking mine. "Your dizziness, is it all of the time or only when you get up from a sitting a lying position?"

"Only when I get up in a hurry. Sometimes I think I'm going to pass out, so I just sit back down again."

"Have you ever had an injury to your neck? This area here." I put my hand on the back of my neck showing where I meant.

She answered no.

Once again she asked me how I knew that she had headaches and dizziness.

"It's because you told me," I answered.

She looked at me even more perplexed.

"How did I tell you? I didn't mention it when I came into the store."

"You're right, you didn't. But then again, you did, but it wasn't orally of course. You told me through what I call 'body language.'"

"This is weird. Just how did my body tell you?"

"By the way you hold your head. You tilt your head from one side to the other, rather than holding it up straight. This told me that you probably have headaches and when I asked you if you did, you answered yes. See, you're doing it again."

"I've never heard that before. Are you saying that just because I tilt my head from side to side, that means I have headaches?"

"No, I'm saying that it's a symptom of a nutritional deficiency. I'm trying to confirm it through additional questioning."

"But that's the way I always hold my head."

"If it's not from an injury, is it just a habit?"

"Can't it just be because I hold my head that way? I've never had a neck or head injury that I'm aware of, unless my mom dropped me as a baby."

"Or unless the doctor had a difficult time in delivering you."

"What does my head have to do with being born?"

"Sometimes during a difficult delivery there could be too much twisting and turning of the baby's head while being extracted from the mother. This is the cause of some neck problems that arise later in life."

"My mom said I was easy compared to my brother. So if I didn't have a neck injury while being born, I guess that I just hold my head this way from habit. Anyway, no one has ever mentioned it before, even the doctor."

"Even the doctor" was a clue that she was at least getting professional help for her condition; whatever it might be.

"Do you have allergies?"

"Yes."

"Do you have tingling in your hands or your legs?"

"Yes."

"Do the bottoms of your feet burn?"

"Yes. Yes."

She was becoming stressed by my questioning. Too easily. It was obvious that she had been deeply stressed for a long time, which had affected her adrenal glands, weakening them to the point of exhaustion. That is why she tilted her head from side to side. It was one of many signals about her adrenal glands.

"Is this going to take any longer? I have to go get my energy pill at another store since I don't see my brand here. Anyway, my vitamin store never mentioned that I have a bad head before and they're a very reputable company."

"Your head isn't bad, it's just that the salespeople at the other stores didn't understand or realize what the significance of holding your head that way could mean. You asked me for an energy pill, which made me curious. So I started looking for reasons why. I suspected your adrenal glands and started asking questions to confirm my suspicion. Weak or exhausted adrenal glands go hand in hand with a lack of energy. And, unfortunately, everyone is selling you energy pills instead of determining why you don't have any energy. It's like putting a Band-Aid on a severed artery. It only helps for a short while and then..."

"And then what?" she asked.

I didn't respond to her question but instead asked her if she had a lot of stress in her life. She nodded her head up and down without looking at me.

"What brought you into this store?"

"I don't know. I had just left the doctor's office and instead of getting into my car I kept on walking. I needed to think."

I knew that the only doctor's office within walking distance was directly across the street from our store. A very busy street. "You just crossed a four-lane road because you wanted to walk." It was a statement rather than a question.

"Yeah, and then I saw your store and I came in to buy my usual energy pills. My regular vitamin store was out of them and I thought, well, maybe you would have them. I really need them. Do have some other brand that's just as good?" she asked as if her resistance was beginning to weaken.

"What was the reason you were seeing the doctor?"

"Depression," she answered somewhat sheepishly.

"Did he put you on medication?"

"Actually he's a she, I mean she's a female doctor. Yes, I'm on several prescription drugs for depression. They just make me drowsy and tired; that's why I need an energy pill."

"How long have you been seeing the doctor for your depression?"

"For about a year. It was right when I started back to school last fall."

"How old are you?"

"Eighteen. Almost nineteen."

Her spontaneous answers told me that she was becoming more comfortable with my questioning, so I decided to get real personal and ask her the really important one. I looked directly into her eyes as I asked her, "How many times have you tried suicide?"

"Twice."

Twice. Her answer rattled in my brain. This so very young woman, only eighteen, had tried suicide twice. What could be so wrong in her life for her to want to end it?

She confided that her parents were getting a divorce and that she left home because of their constant arguing and fighting. She loved them both and felt that maybe it was her fault they were divorcing, even though she eventually found out that there was another person in her father's life.

She quit college and tried living with some friends but they were into drugs, and so she went back to living with her mom after her dad moved out. She wanted to go back to school but had to find a job first to help her mom with the expenses, and her car needed some work. Her whole world seemed to be crashing down on her.

I expected her to be crying about now but there were no tears visible. She was probably doing her crying on the inside, where it hurt the most.

"I want to cry, but I can't."

"What?" I asked. Was she psychic? How did she know I was thinking about tears and crying?

"I want to cry but the tears don't come," she answered. "Sometimes I feel like I'm just going to explode. I mean, it feels as if my heart is going to blow from this body 'cause life, it…it hurts so much."

If my wife had been present she would be hugging this young woman and telling her that everything would be okay. That's why the girl had tried suicide. She only wanted things to get better, both with her parents and herself. I asked her a few more questions about deficiencies and her answers confirmed my suspicions. I walked over to the B vitamin section and took a bottle off the shelf.

"Even if I had the brand of energy pill you were looking for, I would not have sold it to you. This is what you need. This is what your body is deficient in and that's why your body is giving you all those symptoms." I showed her the bottle.

"How much does it cost?" she asked.

"The cost is immaterial. It's the benefit derived from it that is more important. But to answer your question, it's about one-fourth less than the cost of your energy pill and you will probably take a lot fewer of them."

"What is pan...panto...pantotheenic acid, and what does it mean by 'acid'?"

"It's vitamin B-5 and it's pronounced pan-to-then-ic acid. But you were close enough. It's known as the anti-stress vitamin, and the deficiency symptoms of this vitamin are what your body displayed and your answers verified. Pantothenic acid is essential to every cell in the body, and if it's lacking it lessens the body's production of cortisone, which is associated with adrenal exhaustion. So your lack of energy is probably adrenal exhaustion."

She took the bottle from my hand and began reading the label. "It doesn't say anywhere that it's for all those things you said."

"It's in the book. Here, I'll show you," I said as I started toward the bookshelf.

"No, that's okay, I trust you."

"I trust you." The words were like sweet music to my ears. "I trust you." She held the bottle to her breast and closed her eyes. She didn't tell me, but I thought she was saying a silent prayer that this vitamin might help her. At least, that was what I was hoping.

We finally introduced ourselves. She said her name was Tricia. I sold Tricia the bottle of pantothenic acid (B-5) and then showed her the Body Language Questionnaire. I told her to take it home, complete it, and bring it back so that I could do a more in-depth evaluation of her deficiencies.

She said she would be back on Saturday.

I never wish time to pass because it is so valuable and irreplaceable, but I was looking forward to Saturday and said a little prayer each night that she would come back so I could see how she was doing.

Saturday did finally arrive and so did Tricia—an almost new Tricia.

"Hi Bob," she called out as she entered the store. "Here's my answer sheet. I answered yes to quite a few questions. Is that good or bad?"

I smiled and said a silent "thank you" for my prayers being answered.

The change is her was truly remarkable. She stood tall and had a positive energy about her. I was seeing good body language, a picture of health.

"Hey, Bob, I took that panto stuff, you know, I took it three, four, and even five times a day. That's not too much is it? I mean I didn't overdose, did I? Anyway, my dizziness is completely gone. Look." With that she bent over, touched her toes with her fingers, as her long hair flowed onto the floor. Then she abruptly stood up straight.

"See, no dizziness at all. That panto stuff is a miracle drug. I mean vitamin. Oh, I know I'm just jabbering, but honestly, Bob, I'm feeling so much better. I can't believe it. I've been taking all kinds of prescribed drugs these past few months, some for pain, some for energy, and some for depression. You sell me one vitamin pill and all those problems are almost gone, and in less than a week. Wow."

"And what about the headaches?" I asked.

"They're gone too. Well, almost. If I feel one coming on, I just take a panto pill and even a second one an hour or so later, and then the headache disappears. It's really a miracle pill; I even have my mom taking it. That's okay, isn't it? I mean she said it's helping her, so I figured it would be okay for her. After all, she's older than me so it must be safe for her too. Boy, I'm really babbling at the mouth, but I'm so much happier than when I first saw you. And I don't need the energy pill anymore. You were right about that too."

I told Tricia that even though pantothenic acid is not an energy pill, it feeds the adrenal glands in order to strengthen them. This would enable her body to combat stress more readily, and thus she would have more energy.

When she finally settled down, we went over her completed Body Language Questionnaire. She answered many of the almost 300 questions on this questionnaire, which again confirmed one thing: if a person is deficient in one supplement, he or she is usually deficient in others.

Her answer sheet told me she was deficient in most of the minerals, especially magnesium and calcium. They are both instrumental in alleviating stress. This deficiency was also probably why her shoulders were slumped over and why she had menstrual cramping.

"Good, now I know why I have these problems. Let's go for it. Did I tell you I have a job? So sell me what I need."

Thirty-eight dollars and some change later Tricia took her new supplements, shook my hand, and promised she would keep in touch. Thirty eight dollars to change her life.

A couple of months later I received a phone call from her.

"Bob, listen."

There was silence.

"Listen to what?" I asked.

"Wait. I have to get closer 'cause we don't have a portable phone yet."

Again I waited.

"Did you hear it, did you?" she asked excitedly.

"Hear what?" I asked.

"Didn't you hear anything?"

"Yes, I heard what sounded like the flushing of a toilet, but I don't think I want to know why you wanted me to hear you flushing a toilet."

"But I do. I wanted you to be the first to know it, besides me of course."

I was afraid to ask, "First to know about what?" but I finally did.

"Bob, I truly feel I'm all better. That's why I just flushed all my prescription drugs down the toilet, and I wanted to share my excitement with you."

Between her laughing and crying she also told me that her mother was doing better and that she was going to bring her in to see me for nutritional counseling. Tricia was back to school, doing well at her job, but most of all, most of all, she said, "Life doesn't hurt anymore."

Her confidence had improved so much that she decided to enter our local beauty pageant and compete for Miss Santa Clarita Valley. Did she win? Actually, Tricia has been winning every day since she first entered my store. All of this, just because she tilted her head from side to side and I wouldn't sell her an energy pill.

I often think of Tricia, especially in writing this book, and wonder if she would have tried suicide the third time. Perhaps the final time. What influence brought her into my store? What if I had had the brand of energy pill she wanted, would she have been as receptive to my questioning?

Yes, Tricia, I think of you often and am glad I was able to touch your life.

I learned about the tilting of one's head from Neva Jensen, a master herbalist with whom I worked for several years. She said, "Bob, the body tells us when we're hurting, when we're feeling better, and when we're well. I believe that it also tells us when we're about to get sick or when the body becomes diseased. Look at people. Look into their eyes, look past their eyes, watch how they move, stand, or sit. Look for those little things that tell you more about them than what they say."

10

I'M NOT SCHIZOID

"Can I use your bathroom again?" asked Judy, the nineteen-year-old daughter of my customer, Terry.

"Of course. You know where it is, there's no need for someone to show you the way." I looked at Terry and asked, "Does Judy have a bladder infection?"

"No, she has loose bowels," said Terry, somewhat disgustedly.

"How long has she had this problem?" I asked.

"It comes and goes. This time, she's had it for about a month. The doctor thinks she might be schizoid. He believes she brings it on to get attention."

"I can think of better ways to gain attention than feigning diarrhea," I responded. "Although I don't know your daughter that well, she appears to be a rather warm and friendly person. Do you and she have a good mother-daughter relationship?"

"We're the best of buddies. And yes, Judy is a warm and friendly person with lots of friends."

"Those are positive signs. Does the doctor really believe she has a mental disorder? Is she being treated for schizophrenia?"

"He's not sure, and, consequently, she is not being treated. He wants me to take her to a psychiatrist, but psychiatry is not covered under our insurance policy. Also, I'm embarrassed to say, we really can't afford one. We're thinking of selling my car to pay for the testing and subsequent appointments. Yes, Bob, we're in a financial predicament—another reason we pulled Judy out of college. Her impending illness has consumed much of her college tuition."

About that time Judy reappeared, looking pale. I asked her if she needed a glass of water, and she answered that she did. Because of the frequent diarrhea, I offered her a glass of water combined with Emergen-C. This drink would provide her with the electrolyte minerals that are usually lost with her bowel problem. As she took the cup from me I noticed a rash on her neck.

"Judy, before you take a drink, let me see your tongue."

"What? My tongue?"

"Yes, your tongue." I said it somewhat sternly. She extended her tongue just long enough for me to see the redness of it.

"Is your tongue always so red?" I asked. She answered in the affirmative.

"What's the matter with her tongue?" asked Terry.

I ignored her mother's question and asked Judy if she had difficulty reading. Specifically, did the words seem to move as she was reading?

"That's a strange question. No, they don't. But sometimes when I look at myself in the mirror, I see my face changing. That's why the doctor said I might have a tendency toward schizophrenia. I guess he thinks I'm nuts."

"Or very deficient in niacin," I chimed in.

"What's niacin, and what does that have to do with schizophrenia?" asked Terry.

Once again I ignored Judy's mother and continued questioning Judy.

"How long have you had that rash on your neck?"

Judy reached for the collar of her blouse, realizing that it was not covering the rash.

"Oh, this? I've had it for several months now. The doctor said the rash is the least of my worries. However, he did give me a hydrocortisone cream to apply."

"Doesn't work, does it?" I asked.

"It's obvious that you already know the answer. Does the rash have anything to do with my other problems or is it, as the doctor said, 'the least of my worries'?"

"Judy, I want you to make the time to take a Body Language Questionnaire. Hopefully, your answers will confirm my suspicion that you are very deficient in vitamin B-3. This vitamin is more commonly known as niacin or niacinamide. The doctors refer to it as nicotinic acid or nicotinamide. Whatever one calls it, it's basically the same."

"How can she be deficient in this vitamin? She takes vitamins. I know, I send them, or used to send them to her at college."

I looked at Judy.

"Mom, they made me sick, so I never took them."

"And being at college, you probably never had time for food, good food. The vitamins made you sick because you took them either on an empty stomach or with a limited amount of liquid," I added.

Judy's sheepish look verified my statement.

"Judy, how could you?" asked her mother.

Before Judy could answer, I interjected. "Terry, it's not what she did or didn't do. What's important is what you and Judy do now. If my suspicions are correct, Judy's problems could be corrected for less than ten dollars, that is, if she takes her suggested vitamins and you do the cooking for her until she's ready to go back to college."

"How can you be so sure that it's a vitamin deficiency?"

"Ladies, niacin has a reputation for correcting the three D's—dermatitis, diarrhea, and dementia. I realized Judy might have a deficiency when I saw her rash, her red tongue, and heard that she has vision problems. All these symptoms relate to a deficiency in niacin. That's why I want Judy to do the questionnaire to confirm my belief."

Judy's answers to the Body Language Questionnaire indicated that she was extremely deficient in the B vitamins, especially niacin. After several weeks of Mom's cooking and Judy's taking the suggested supplements, she was able to return to college for the following semester. The lesser cost of the supplements, versus the doctor bills, enabled the family to afford the college tuition once again.

11

VITAMIN A AND THE BIRTH OF A CHILD

Beverly came into the store a little after noon. I noted that she was wearing sunglasses even though there was only a limited amount of sunshine, no glare, and lots of clouds. We exchanged greetings, and I asked how I could help her.

"Bob, I just need some vitamin C. In capsules please, and, yes, I'll take two of the large bottles. We go through them so fast."

I got her two bottles of vitamin C and proceeded to the check stand to register her purchase. In any other retail store, this might be considered a normal purchase. The customer makes her request, the item is retrieved, rung up on the cash register, placed in a bag, paid for, and the customer leaves. But not in my store. I saw something out of the ordinary that made me suspicious, so I asked a question—a question that ultimately changed the lives of three people.

"Bev, why the sunglasses?"

By asking a question, I was creating a conversation that would eventually result in an exchange of information that could be pertinent to some condition she had.

After asking the question, different thoughts entered my mind. What if her husband had given her a black eye? No, he's a good man; he wouldn't do that, would he? I was almost sorry I had asked, but this was my usual approach to finding out how I could help someone—ask the embarrassing question so that I might be able to help.

Bev looked around the store to confirm that only the two of us were present.

"Only for you, Bob, would I do this," she answered. Then she lifted the glasses onto the top of her head, revealing eyes that were extremely puffy and swollen, especially the upper eyelids.

"Have you been to the doctor?" I asked.

"Yes."

"What did he say it was?"

"He wasn't quite sure, so he is doing some testing to determine the cause."

"Do they burn or itch?" I asked.

"No, they're just swollen. I wake up in the morning with them this way, and even with prescription eyedrops they are not getting any better. Bob, do you have any ideas?" she asked pleadingly.

"Bev, let me see the back of your arms," I asked.

"The back of my arms? What for? It's the eyes that I asked you about," she said almost sarcastically.

"Yes, the back of your arms. I need to confirm a suspicion."

She rolled back the sleeves of her blouse, enabling me to see the back of her arms. Both of them had a huge area of goose bumps that looked like pimples. I then asked her if she had any sinus problems.

"Yes," came her answer.

"Do you catch cold easily?"

"Yes."

"Bev, it looks as if you are extremely deficient in vitamin A. Your body is telling me with the pimples on your arms, the puffiness of your eyelids, the sinus problems, and the catching cold easily. These are all symptoms of a deficiency of this particular vitamin."

"I can't take vitamin A," was her answer.

"Why? Are you allergic to it?" I asked, knowing her answer had to be *no.*

"I'm trying to get pregnant, and the doctor said I should stay away from anything that had vitamin A in it. He said it causes birth defects."

"How long have you been trying, as you put it, to get pregnant?" I asked.

"Bob, I'm thirty-eight years old. I, we, have been trying to get pregnant for five years now without any success. We want a child so badly before I'm too old to conceive and deliver."

"How many miscarriages have you had?" I assumed that she had at least one.

"Four. I've been pregnant four times for a total of eight months. I lose the baby after two months. They don't know why. I guess we weren't supposed to have a child."

"And the doctor said you are to stay away from vitamin A," I repeated.

Her answer was once again *yes.*

"Bev, I know you're on your lunch hour, but we have to talk more about this, and it could take a lot longer than the time you have now."

"If it's about me getting pregnant and carrying full term, I mean—do you believe I might be able to? If so, I'll take an extended lunch hour."

Fortunately my wife, Pat, came into the store to relieve me for lunch, which I willingly forfeited in order to spend some time with Bev.

"Beverly," I began, "let's talk about vitamin A. After we're through with this discussion, I'm going to ask a very big favor of you, a favor that will require both you and your husband to give me the answer I want. But first, with your permission, I want to tell you a story."

Bev nodded her agreement and listened with interest as I related an experience that occurred years ago when I was just starting out in the nutrition industry.

I had been in the business only a few months when a woman who was probably in her late fifties approached me. I didn't realize it until she told me her story as to why her skin looked so soft and supple. She was almost wrinkle-free. She asked me where the vitamin A section was located, so I guided her accordingly and asked what potency she wanted. She asked if vitamin A was available in liquid form. I said no and that the highest potency was 25,000 iu in a soft gelatin capsule.

She said, somewhat disgustedly, "Then I'll have to keep taking twelve of these a day."

I did a quick calculation and said to her, "Why, ma'am, that's 300,000 units. You shouldn't be taking that much vitamin A."

"Why?" she asked. "Can it be dangerous?"

Even though I was very new in the industry I had been doing a lot of research and reading, and I also had been a pharmaceutical salesman for over four years. Most researchers, especially those in the medical profession, agreed that this oil-soluble vitamin, when taken in excessive amounts, is not readily and harmlessly excreted, as in the case of vitamins C and B. Instead, vitamin A can build up in the liver with harmful consequences and eventually become toxic.

"Honey," she asked in a superior tone, "what are the symptoms of too much vitamin A?"

I answered, "Intermittent joint pain, fatigue, weight loss, hair loss, and even death."

"Hair loss?" she asked. "You mean like this?" and she reached for her hair and, much to my shock, removed a wig from her head, revealing a very bald scalp. I was flabbergasted. I couldn't say a word. That's when she started laughing at me.

"Honey, I have been taking this much vitamin A for over eight years. I was seventy-two years old when I was told I had less than six months to live because of bladder cancer and I should prepare for my inevitable demise. That's when I started mega-vitamin therapy by taking lots of vitamin A with lots of vitamins E and C to lessen any negative effect of a possible A overdose. The loss of my hair was caused by chemotherapy and radiation, not from an overdose of vitamin A. I've been teasing you, honey, and if you could have seen the look on your face when I pulled off my wig—it was hilarious."

This woman, whom I believed to be in her late fifties, was almost eighty years old and yet she had the skin of a much younger person. Even her eyes were a clear, light blue. It was so apparent that vitamin A, a skin and eye vitamin, was doing wonders both in maintaining this woman's health and enabling her to look younger.

Bev was smiling at the story I had just told her.

"So you see, Bev, vitamin A could be toxic, but this woman took precautions when she took that much. The extra vitamin E and C both increased the effectiveness of vitamin A and protected her from overdosing on it. She also told me that she sometimes would stop taking that high an amount for up to three or fours days. This allowed her liver to excrete any excess. In fact, many researchers state that the liver can absorb and store at least 500,000 iu of this vitamin. That doesn't mean you can or should take that much, but if you were to the antidote is simple. If symptoms of an overdose occur, merely reduce the intake of the vitamin or stop it for a few days."

"So you're saying that I should be taking vitamin A even though the doctor said to stay away from it?" she asked.

"No, Bev, I never tell anyone to not take a doctor's prescription or to not listen to their professional advice. I tell a story and explain the nutrient, and then it's up to the customer to reach his or her own conclusion."

She said, "Well, based on this story, I should be taking vitamin A. What about the birth defects that it causes? Shouldn't that be a consideration?"

"Bev, allow me to continue about vitamin A and its importance in the human body and how it relates to pregnancy. Incidentally," I asked, "did you know that vitamin A is referred to as the growth vitamin?" She shook her head no. I continued. "Many children throughout the world and even the United States suffer from stunted growth because of a deficiency of vitamin A. Why do you suppose that children grow faster or taller in the summer months than the in winter months? Do you think it could be that vitamin A is more readily available in the summer?" I didn't want to overwhelm Bev with too much information, but I needed her to realize the importance of this vitamin.

"Did you know that a worldwide deficiency of vitamin A causes permanent blindness in tens of thousands of children?"

Again she shook her head no and asked, "Why is there so much negativity about this vitamin?"

"It probably started before the early 1940s and the introduction of penicillin and other antibiotics. Vitamin A, no, synthetic vitamin A, was the therapy of choice for lung diseases such as whooping cough and pneumonia. Imagine a young mother holding her sick baby who was gasping for breath. The prescribed therapy was vitamin A, maybe one or two drops a day. But this young mother believed that if one or two drops were good, perhaps ten or more drops would be better. She was desperate, and being a loving mother, of course, increased her child's dose without realizing she was doing more harm by increasing the doctor's prescribed recommendation. How much was she giving? Did she stop at ten drops, or was fifteen or even twenty better? Yes, in many cases the child would die and it was blamed on an overdose of vitamin A. This holds true to this day. Instead of saying that excessive amounts of vitamin A are dangerous, it has been changed over the years to just 'vitamin A is toxic' with no reference to the word *excessive.* This outcome is unfortunate because vitamin A plays such an important role in all aspects of the human body.

"Vitamin A prevents infectious diseases. In your case, your swollen eyes indicate a lack of A, as do your skin, lungs, and, of course, your inability to carry a child to term. All these parts of your body are competing for vitamin A, but obviously your liver's store of this vitamin has been depleted. Now you have been told to stay away from this vitamin because of its toxicity. Your deficiency symptoms are so very, very obvious, and it's a shame that vitamin A has received such an inaccurate reputation.

"Vitamin A is found in all mucous membranes of the body, including the eyes, lungs, alimentary canal, and in all organs of the body including the heart and reproductive organs. It helps your body ward off infection by promoting the growth of mucous in the mucous membrane lining. If you have little or no vitamin A, the linings of these tracts become keratinized. Instead of normal healthy cells, which secrete mucous, the cells become hard, dry, and scaly. Thus a sperm and egg are unable to niche onto the uterus as the keratinization process becomes a barrier. Consequently, the sperm and egg are sloughed off. Additionally, vitamin A determines the depth of a child's gender. By depth, I mean all boy or all girl. Do you think it's possible that the diminished intake of vitamin A by prospective parents over the past fifty years could increase the possibility of homosexuality?

"Bev, has anyone, including your doctor, told you that a lack of vitamin A causes birth defects including cleft palate, defects of the heart and eyes including anophthalmos, which is a child born without eyes? Probably not, as some medical people emphasize only the negative effects of vitamin A. And now, Bev, as I said earlier, I want to ask a big favor of you, which will also require your husband's input as well. Are you ready?"

She looked at me, perhaps wondering what I might ask next. After a few moments of silence, she answered, "Bob, I have known you for several years. I know you are a man of your word and I do wholeheartedly trust you. Ask me the favor. I will discuss it with Jack and we'll give you our answer by tomorrow. What is it that you are asking?"

"I want you to forget about getting pregnant for at least four and possibly six months." She had a perplexed look on her face; perhaps it was anguish. Before she could ask why, I continued.

"Please consider mega-vitamin therapy for a few months to correct your vitamin A deficiency. There are some nutritional doctors who recommend up to 100,000 iu a day with additional E and C. Continue with this program until your obvious deficiency symptoms disappear. I will also ask that you complete a Body Language Questionnaire to determine if you have any other short supply of nutrients. Additionally, take 400 units of vitamin E plus extra pantothenic acid to prevent or, at the least, lessen any stretch marks when you do get pregnant. Bev, as your friend, please consider these requests."

I didn't have to wait until the next day for their answer. They both came back to the store within the hour and agreed to my requests.

The four of us—Bev, Jack, I, and their son, who is now over twenty-four years old—are so pleased with their decision. All because of a pair of sunglasses and an embarrassing little question.

Oh, I should also add that their son is over six feet tall—much taller than his father. Perhaps it's because vitamin A, which is known as the growth vitamin, works.

12

ICHTHYOSIS

Sweet sixteen, sweet seventeen, sweet eighteen—and still she had never been kissed. Well...she'd been kissed, but only by her parents, her dog, and a few relatives. But she had never been kissed directly on the lips. Oh, she wanted to be kissed, but no one wanted to kiss her—they didn't dare because of her problem. She had cried herself to sleep countless times asking the usual question, "Why me?" Although she herself had never been kissed, she had been doing the kissing herself. At the age of twelve she learned about kissing from her older sister, Beth. The two of them would discuss Beth's date from the previous evening and how she was kissed goodnight.

"Will anyone ever kiss me?" she would ask her sister, who then reassured her that someday it would happen. And throughout the next six years, her kisses had been limited to the kissing of her doll, her teddy bear, and even her own hand. She would put her forefinger and thumb together and pretend they were the lips of her knight in shining armor.

Her dad blamed her for her dilemma.

"If you would keep a handkerchief or tissue handy, you wouldn't have this problem," he would tell her. Yes, she had always suffered from allergies, which caused her nose to run, but she always used a tissue. It was not her fault. Even the doctors were stymied.

Laurel was a school friend of my daughter. They had several classes together, ate lunch at the same time, and rode home from school in the same bus. When Laurel would accompany my daughter to our home, it would be when my wife and I were at work. Although I knew who Laurel was by name, I never met her. At her request, my daughter never discussed Laurel's affliction with me. She was afraid that if my wife and I knew of her ailment, we wouldn't allow our daughter to continue their friendship. My daughter couldn't convince her otherwise.

It wasn't until the day before graduation that I came home from work early and finally met Laurel. She was obviously embarrassed when I walked into the kitchen where she and my daughter were preparing an after school snack and discussing the prom, which Laurel had missed. She wanted to go, but no one had asked her.

She was very attractive, with long, light brown hair, a slight build, and friendly blue eyes. Why had she not been asked to the prom? For the same reason she had never been kissed. Its medical name is Ichthyosis.

This disease is characterized by dryness, harshness, and scaly-ness of the skin. It has an eczema-like appearance and is commonly referred to as "fish scales." It usually occurs around the hair follicles, but in Laurel's case it encompassed her mouth.

When my daughter introduced us I couldn't help noticing Laurel's problem, and I could also tell that she had become very embarrassed.

"I have to go now," she said to my daughter.

"But we haven't eaten yet. You can't go. You promised to stay until four o'clock."

Laurel turned away and started toward the door, saying over her shoulder that she was glad to meet me.

"Is it chapped lips?" I asked, knowing that the condition was much worse.

"No, it has something to do with a congenital abnormality of the skin," she answered as she continued toward the door.

I persisted. "Is it Ichthyosis?"

She stopped and turned around immediately, with a surprised look about her.

"Yes, but how do you know, I mean how did you know about this kind of disease?" She looked at my daughter as if to say, "You promised not to tell your parents."

My daughter said, "My dad knows about these things. I didn't tell him, he just knew."

I spoke up. "Laurel, I used to be in the pharmaceutical industry and I sold products for various skin conditions. I've seen several cases of Ichthyosis, but it mostly occurs in the hair line."

"Yeah, I got lucky, didn't I? I got it where it's most noticed," she said in a half-sarcastic, half-pathetic way.

"Are they doing the usual therapy for you?"

"Yes, if you mean the usual cortisone."

I nodded.

"Sometimes it works for a little while, but most of the time I look like this. Actually it's a little worse than usual today."

My daughter grinned when I kept asking questions. She knew that Laurel's condition had aroused my curiosity and now good old Dad was going to work.

"Laurel, do you also have sinus problems or allergies?"

"Yes, in fact my dad says that my skin problem is caused because of my dripping nose. But I use a tissue all of the time."

I continued, "May I see the back of your arm?"

She looked at my daughter, who reassured her that Dad knew what he was doing.

"I guess I'm getting scaly skin on my arms, too. In fact, I even have these little pimples or bumps on my legs."

"Do you catch colds easily, at least four or more a year?" I asked.

"I guess so. Mostly I get a lot of chest colds and ear infections."

"Laurel, is it possible for you and your mother to visit with me at my store? There's a good possibility that your condition can be lessened considerably, but I need to talk about it with one or both of your parents. Or, if you like, you could come back here with them later on, say, after dinner."

Laurel did come back to our home later on that evening with her mother. I explained to them that Laurel had many symptoms of a vitamin A deficiency and perhaps even vitamin F, which is found in safflower oil. (In those days we didn't have flax, soy, evening primrose oil, or even Emu oil. Only a limited supply of herbs was readily available.)

Her mother looked at Laurel and saw those sweet but hurting blue eyes. They seemed to be saying, "Please, Mommy, let's try it. Let's try it." Even though it was now past nine o'clock and the store was closed, we all agreed that we might as well start the regimen tonight. Together we reopened the store, and they made their purchase of vitamins A, C, E, zinc, lecithin, and safflower oil capsules.

Several weeks later I came home from work and was surprised to see Laurel. She and my daughter had spent the day together, and Laurel wanted to stay until I got home. She wanted to show me what she called her new face. She had convinced her mother, through diligent reading of several nutrition books, to allow her to take 100,000 units of vitamin A each day for the past month. Her mother was worried about an overdose, but the writings of Paavo Airola and James Balch, M.D., had convinced her otherwise.

"Look
I'm almost kissable."

By October, after just a few weeks in junior college, Laurel was dating and, I presume, perhaps even kissing. Why waste six years of practice? Her condition did not return over the next four years. Last I heard, Laurel was moving to Colorado to continue her education.

13

Acne

Oh, how I remember those days of being in high school. I would get up in the morning, look in the mirror, and check to see if any new pimples, or how many, had sprouted up during the night. Unfortunately, newly found pimples sometimes affected my day. My pimples were disgusting and embarrassing, and no one seemed to have a solution to the problem.

Since entering the nutrition industry, I have learned to modify and sometimes correct the problem of adolescent acne. It is with great care and diligence that I approach someone who has this problem. But I do approach him or her because that's what I do—I help others if their condition is nutritionally related.

If I come upon someone not in my store, my usual approach is to say, "I know it's none of my business, but consider talking to someone at a vitamin store about using these supplements. They do work; they worked for my children." I then hand them a paper with the names of several vitamins and the amounts that have been suggested by Dr. John Heinerman, a master herbalist and nutritional counselor.

Sometimes the teenager is receptive and thanks me for my concern. Sometimes he or she gets angry and tells me it's none of my business. However, I don't give up, and I give them this response: "No it's not, and yes it is."

This answer takes them aback for just a moment, enabling me to add, "I suffered for years, enough for both of us. Here's the answer." I offer the note to them again. Sometimes they accept it, and sometimes they don't.

The note usually reads: Talk to a vitamin store nutritional counselor about vitamin A, zinc, the B-complex, and vitamin C.

I also include the amount of vitamin A suggested by Dr. Heinerman and other nutritionists: 100,000 units of vitamin A each day for one month, stop for one week, and resume the vitamin. Do this for three months maximum.

My children can attest to the efficacy of this regimen. After two months, two of them were clear of acne throughout high school. My younger daughter had to repeat the program the following semester before correcting her problem. They took more supplements than I listed above, as do the teenagers who are my customers. At the store, I go into much more detail including diet, bowel movements, cleanliness, etc. The additional supplements are predicated by the results of their Body Language Questionnaire.

Throughout the years it was extremely rewarding when a teenager who had acne problems came into the store and gave me either a hug or a warm handshake because his or her acne condition had either improved tremendously or had totally cleared up. And if the problem ever came back, he or she knew what to do about it.

14

ACNE ON THE FOREHEAD

Even though her bangs were down to her eyebrows, the acne on her forehead was still visible. I'm glad this teenager was in my store with her mother because in that setting, I was able to ask more in-depth, and sometimes personal, questions. I greeted them both and immediately directed my questioning to the young lady.

"Are you being treated for the acne on your forehead?" I asked, knowing the question would take her by surprise. Her mother, however, smiled. She knew I was both honest and direct.

"Yes. I'm seeing a doctor, and a dermatologist, but...nothing seems to work."

I could feel the stress in her voice. She asked me if there was something I could suggest for her to take. She referred to the acne on her forehead as "whiteheads." Marissa had been suffering from this type of acne since school started, and, although she was seeing a dermatologist, her condition was worsening.

"Do you wear contacts?" I asked.

"No," she answered quizzically. "Anyway, what do my eyes have to do with acne?"

Instead of answering, I asked if she had excessive oil in the T-factor of her face.

"Oh, my gosh, yes, I do. That's another thing my doctor was trying to correct, although he blamed it on my heritage and said I would just have to live with it. He also said that many of his patients have the same condition, but they, too, are of the same heritage as me. Oh, my gosh, is it related to my whiteheads? Is that why you asked about my eyes? Do my red eyes have something to do with it? My mom said they were from lack of sleep, because I have so much homework and I stay up so late. Oh please, please, can you do something about that too?"

This bright young teenager was asking questions so fast that I could hardly keep up with her, but finally she stopped rattling on and I started asking her more questions. Her mother's optometrist had prescribed eye drops for Marissa's red, dry eyes, and although they did help, the problem was not corrected. I also determined that she had less than adequate eating habits and poor bowel movements, she consumed too many soft drinks, had improper skin cleansing, and worried too much. Yes, she was stressed-out, too much for anyone. She had asked the proper people for help but, unfortunately, they were not familiar with nutrient deficiencies.

Her vitamin B-2 deficiency was apparent, and yet none of her doctors was treating the cause, just the symptoms. Her mother purchased vitamin B-2, vitamin A, a multiple vitamin, and pantothenic acid, the anti-stress vitamin. Marissa took home the Body Language Questionnaire and returned it the next day for evaluation. She was a changed little girl since the previous day. Now she had hope in her heart that she would be doing better soon. And she was. Her acne problem, eye problems, and oily skin problems cleared up dramatically in less than a month. Within two months, all of her symptoms were corrected.

If only I had known about these supplements when I was in high school.

15

Mouth - Sores at the Corner

Ray, a local realtor, visited my store one day to ask me about the little sores his wife had at the corners of her mouth. He wasn't a believer in nutrition, but sometimes he would venture in and ask my opinion to compare it to what he had read in a medical journal.

I asked if his wife's sores were on the lips or actually at the corners of her mouth.

"The corners," he replied.

"How long has she had them?" I asked.

"Let's see. It's been well over two, no, three months now."

"What did your family doctor diagnose and eventually prescribe?" I asked.

"He thought it was a fungal infection and prescribed an ointment, but that didn't work. At the next appointment he prescribed a cream. That didn't work either, but I think it was because my wife kept licking at the sore and washing the cream off. At this point, our doctor suggested we see a dermatologist. After two appointments and two prescriptions for ointments, which didn't work, the dermatologist recommended we see an allergist. We were supposed to see him this week, but we're going on vacation for two weeks, so I guess we'll have to get one of these other prescriptions refilled."

"Even though they didn't work?" I asked.

"Don't know what else to do. Unless..." he said as more of a question than a statement.

"Unless it can be related to a vitamin deficiency. Is that what you were going to ask?" I proposed.

"Is it possible?"

I asked him a series of questions regarding his wife's condition: "Does she have cataracts? Are her eyes often bloodshot or red? Do her eyes burn, are they dry, do they itch? If it were you, Ray, who had the problem, I would ask if your urine is always a bright yellow or is it pale or even less than pale."

"My wife has all of those things, even the start of cataracts. What is it going to cost me to make her well? Do I have to buy the whole store?"

"Let's see, what have you spent so far? Your wife had three appointments with your regular doctor and two with the dermatologist, plus four prescriptions that didn't work. What would you say those appointments and prescriptions cost you? Based on your answers to my questions about her condition, your wife is deficient in vitamin B-2, also know as riboflavin. This vitamin costs less than five dollars a bottle, and one bottle should be sufficient. However, she should also be taking her multiple vitamin. What else can I help you with?"

Ray and his wife cancelled their appointment with the allergist, went on their two-week vacation, and came from the airport directly to my store to thank me for the vitamin B-2, that little yellow vitamin.

16

MOUTH SORES AND THE DOCTOR

When I had my vitamin stores I lectured on nutrition at local clubs, including the Chamber of Commerce and other community groups.

At one luncheon, I had not been forewarned that there was a very arrogant medical doctor in the audience. As I was lecturing I noticed that one audience member had huge, red sores at the corners of his mouth. I ignored them, of course, as I didn't want to embarrass him in front of his peers. I planned to see him after the meeting to discuss his possible deficiency of vitamin B-2.

At the conclusion of the lecture I asked if there were any questions. The gentleman with the sores at the corners of his mouth was the first to put forth a question.

"Hey, Bob, I have these sores in the corner of my mouth. What do you suggest I take to correct this problem?"

If I had answered his question directly, it would have been considered diagnosing and prescribing. That's something I never do because I am not licensed to practice medicine. Instead, I asked him if he wanted to discuss it after the meeting.

"No," he replied, "you're the expert. Tell me what to do."

So I asked him, in front of his peers, the usual questions related to a deficiency of vitamin B-2. I thought that if I embarrassed him it would be because of his own persistence. His answers indicated that he was deficient in many of the B vitamins. I suggested that he consider a multiple vitamin, and that, if he wanted, he could temporarily take some additional B-2. He wrote down the names of the vitamins, thanked me, and said he would get them after work. I thought it all went well.

Suddenly, I was interrupted by the doctor, his doctor, the one who had been unsuccessful in treating his problem. "I am a medical doctor, and what you just diagnosed as a deficiency of a vitamin is called..."

I didn't quite understand the medical term he used, but he was obviously upset. I started to defend myself, saying that I didn't diagnose.

He continued. "Your crackpot industry is trying to play doctor without a license. Your whole industry should be investigated."

I had unintentionally stepped on his toes, so I decided it was time to end my lecture.

"Ladies and gentlemen. I always record my own lectures. If any of you would like a copy, please let me know."

I thanked them and proceeded to pack up my papers and leave. I don't usually offer the recording of my lectures to anyone, but I wanted to make the doctor aware that I had recorded proof that I did not diagnose or prescribe.

Later that day, I received several telephone calls from members of the club, all apologizing for the doctor's comments. It was apparent to them that he was embarrassed by his inability to correct his patient's vitamin B-2 deficiency through the usual medical treatments.

His patient visited my store, bought the suggested vitamins, and called three weeks later to say his condition was corrected.

Another story...

Frank was and still is a movie actor. Even after many years, I occasionally still see him on television, only now he plays the part of a respectful older gentleman. Where have the years gone?

Frank came into the store early one afternoon, and after our mutual greetings I asked him why he was taking so much vitamin B-6.

"How did you know I'm taking B-6?" he asked.

"Because you have created a deficiency of vitamin B-2," I countered. I knew that Frank was faithful in taking his multiple vitamin, but I also knew that he experimented with supplements a lot.

Frank had been on location in Hawaii for the past two months and had gained several unneeded pounds because of the rich, good food. In fact, according to his director, he was fat. Frank knew that B-6 was a good diuretic, so he began taking excess doses of B-6 without increasing any of the complementing B vitamins. He developed sores in the corners of his mouth, which, as you now know, is a visual sign of a B-2 deficiency. He said that the makeup artist was going crazy trying to cover these open sores, but to no avail. Each time Frank would laugh or cry out according to the requirements of the script, it caused his mouth to extend wider than usual, revealing his two sores through all of the makeup.

I suggested he take additional B-2 for a few weeks and consider increasing the dosage of his multivitamin to two or three a day until the sores healed.

"We could use you on the set to correct all of our problems," he said one day.

Unfortunately, I never got that opportunity, but Frank's problem sores disappeared, much to his and his makeup artist's and director's delight.

17

EYES - CAN'T SEE IN DIM LIGHT

There are times when a statement or word arouses my curiosity. Such was the case one day when the Edison Electric representative came into the store to get a meter reading. I guided him to the back room and showed him the meter.

He thanked me for being so courteous and then added that the "bar people" weren't as friendly as me (one of my stores was a couple of doors down from a beer bar). "It's hard to see in there. It's so dark that it takes a few minutes for my eyes to adjust before I can even make out the meter."

Okay, he made a comment about a bar that offers limited lighting. I've been told that most bars are dark inside. I don't know why, but they are, so? Nevertheless, his comment prompted a question from me, in fact, several questions.

"Do you catch cold easily?" I asked.

"Yes, why do you ask?" he responded.

I ignored his question and continued with mine.

"Do have difficulty seeing at night?"

"Yes," he replied.

"Do you have little goose bumps on the back of your arms or on the top of your legs?"

"Yes. Yes I do," he said, a surprised look on his face.

"Do you have sinus problems?"

And, of course, I received another *yes* from him. His answers convinced me that he had a deficiency in vitamin A. He said he'd had respiratory problems all of his life, or at least as long as he could remember. Yes, they took out his tonsils thinking that this would cure him of his ills. It didn't, of course.

I explained the benefits of vitamin A, and he bought a small bottle. At my further suggestion he bought some vitamin C, E, and a multiple vitamin. I gave him a Body Language Questionnaire to fill out at home. His parting words?

"Wow, thanks. I'm feeling better already."

He probably did, but only because he found a salesperson who cared—cared about him and his health and asked the right questions. A few weeks later he visited my store to tell me of his excellent progress.

18

NIGHT VISION

"Why don't you drive the last few miles home?" Don suggested.

"Sure, I'd be glad to," I answered.

For the last several fishing trips, I had been asked by my friend to do the driving. I enjoy driving, as does he, but why was he asking me to do the driving for him? I didn't think he was sleepy. The last two times I had driven for him, he stayed awake. He didn't even try to doze, not even slightly.

Don knows I do nutritional counseling, but he has never asked my opinion or inquired about my profession. And I don't ever push a friend or relative into a conversation about their health. I had to ease into a discussion with Don that would eventually tell me the reason he didn't want to drive. We had both slept during the return trip of our fishing boat, so I wasn't sleepy, and I presumed that he wasn't either. As I was running this perplexing problem through my mind, an oncoming car approached with its high beams on. I blinked my lights and commented, "Wow. They were sure bright lights."

"You too?" Don asked.

"What do you mean, 'you too'?" I asked in response to his question.

"Do those headlights bother you too?"

Dimness of vision at night is a common cause of vehicular accidents, and vitamin A plays a monumental role in correcting this problem. I asked Don a few questions to determine the extent of his deficiency of this vitamin.

"Do you catch cold easily? Do you have sinus problems? Do you have ear infections? Do you have goose-bump-like pimples on the back of your arm? Do your eyes tire very easily? Are your eyes often red? Does mucous accumulate around your eyes, especially at night? Do you ever have sores at the corners of your mouth?"

As one of his best friends, certainly his best fishing buddy, I should have been aware if any of these conditions applied to him. Even among the best of friends not all things are discussed, particularly when it comes to health. Fortunately, Don adopted a trusting attitude and became very frank with me. He admitted to answering many *yeses* to a vitamin A deficiency, but he did not answer yes to the questions relating to a vitamin B-2 deficiency. Vitamin B-2 can also play a role in the health of the eyes, but Don did not appear deficient in this vitamin.

After we had driven in silence for a while, he asked if I would be willing to go to my store and sell him a bottle of vitamin A.

19

Vitamin A
Why It Didn't Work for Him

"I tried your vitamin A and it didn't work. I'm still blinded by oncoming headlights."

It had been decided months earlier that Mark's night vision was impaired by the glare of lights, especially headlights. He was extremely deficient in vitamin A; thus it was recommended that he take vitamin A to correct his problem. Obviously, it didn't work.

"How much have you been taking on a daily basis, and have you been taking it daily?"

"Bob, at first I took it just once a day, because I was also getting some in my multivitamin. I didn't want to overdose. After two weeks, I didn't notice any vision improvements. Then someone at work told me to increase the dosage, so I did. I started taking three a day and have been for the last two months. Still no change in my vision and in two months I start working the graveyard shift, which means I have to drive at night. I can't afford to lose my job, or my life. Help me."

Mark was certainly faithful in taking his vitamin A. Why it didn't work for him would have to be determined. Again I asked several questions related to a deficiency of vitamin A, and his answers indicated he was still lacking in this vitamin. Was he assimilating the vitamin?

"Mark, do you have a problem eating spicy foods?"

"Yes, especially when my wife makes her favorite Mexican dish. Why are we talking about food?"

"There is a correlation. What happens when you eat spicy foods? How does your body, or specifically your stomach, tolerate it?"

"It doesn't. I get pain in my side." He pointed to an area to the right and below his rib cage. "And then I feel as if I'm going to throw up. My wife said it was my gallbladder. She should know—she used to have that problem."

"And why doesn't she anymore?" I asked.

"She cleansed it. She took it out of her stomach and brushed it real good and got all of that gravel stuff out of it." He was grinning. Then he got real. "No, she didn't do it that way. She took a concoction of two lemons and two tablespoons of olive oil, mixed them up real good, and drank the stuff. She said it tasted okay, something like a salad dressing. Maybe I should try it."

"Mark, she may be right. You are not assimilating your fat-soluble vitamins—not only vitamin A, but vitamin E as well. Why don't you check with your doctor about your gallbladder? Maybe Maria is right about its being the cause of your pain."

Mark did check with his doctor and found out that he did indeed have a sluggish gallbladder. When he discussed the doctor's diagnosis with Maria, she insisted that he do her gallbladder cleanse. He did it three times over three days and soon was able to eat spicy foods without a problem. In addition, he started taking digestive enzymes and, as a result, began to assimilate vitamin A more effectively.

20

Burns and Not Scarring

Only a mother can feel the hurt in her child when she hears screams of pain. Such was the situation many years ago when a young mother who had been ironing left the room to answer the telephone downstairs. Before she could answer it she heard the mixed screaming of Lisa, her four-year-old daughter, and Adam, her six-year-old son. The mother could tell the difference between the screams. One was of fright; the other was of excruciating pain.

You're probably wondering why a mother would leave a hot iron where her children could gain access to it. That was not the case. To ensure her children would not enter the room, this young mother, Peggy, had closed the door of her bedroom when she went to answer the telephone. Additionally, the children had been told to never enter their parents' bedroom when the door was shut without first knocking. In spite of these many precautions, children sometimes forget when they are playing tag, as was the case with Peggy's children.

Adam was "it" and was chasing after Lisa. Without thinking, and needing a place to hide, Lisa ran into her mother's bedroom even though the door was closed. As she entered her parents' bedroom, Lisa ran directly into the ironing board, knocking her, the ironing board, and the hot iron to the floor. Her right arm landed directly on the hot iron, but it was too hot for her to feel the pain. She let out more of a yell or a yelp because she knew she had done wrong. She thought Mommy would be angry and she might get a spanking. Then she felt the searing heat of the iron against her arm. Her next scream, the one of excruciating pain, startled Peggy.

Peggy raced to the top of the stairs, where she met Adam. He was crying. Through his tears he cried out, "Mommy, Lisa fell on the iron. I didn't push her; she just knocked it over and fell on it. Help her, Mommy, help her."

Peggy ran past Adam and saw Lisa on the floor lying next to the ironing board. Then she saw why Lisa was screaming. Her right arm was on top of the hot iron. Peggy was puzzled. She couldn't understand why Lisa didn't get up. Why didn't she move her arm off the iron? Peggy bent down to help her. That's when she realized why Lisa wasn't able to do it herself. The iron was sticking to her bare skin.

Peggy slowly and carefully removed the iron to keep the least amount of flesh from tearing away. She almost passed out from the smell of burnt skin sticking to the iron, but she had to stay calm. As she picked Lisa up in her arms, she told Adam to run ahead and get the aloe vera juice in the bathroom cupboard. Upon reaching the bathroom, she sat down with Lisa on her lap.

Lisa was screaming hysterically, the severity of the pain having now reached her nervous system. Adam opened the bottle and handed it to his mother. Peggy liberally applied the aloe to Lisa's now-open wound, reassuring her that her arm would stop hurting soon. She did everything she could to hold back her own tears. Afterward, she said that she wanted to scream at the top of her lungs because of the hurt her little daughter was feeling, but she knew she had to stay calm in order to keep her children calm.

As Peggy poured the liquid over Lisa's arm, Lisa looked up at her, and, with tears filling her beautiful brown eyes, said, "Mommy, it hardly hurts anymore."

Peggy, her husband, Bill, and their two children lived in a rural community where the closest hospital was two hours away and that was by way of an ambulance with flashing red lights and blaring siren. In this situation, Peggy opted to give Lisa first aid herself.

First, she needed a bandage for Lisa's arm and asked Adam to continue applying the aloe while she looked in their medicine cabinet. After soaking the bandage with the aloe, she placed it on Lisa's arm and went back to the bathroom cabinet for some additional things. Powdered calcium, pantothenic acid, and Emergen-C were the three supplements this family had always taken with them on hikes, fishing trips, and camping outings. Calcium lessens the chance of shock and promotes the coagulation of blood to an injured area. Pantothenic acid, known as the anti-stress vitamin, helps the adrenal glands to combat stress, such as caused by the hot iron. Emergen-C provides vitamin C and necessary minerals, especially potassium, all in a packet form, enabling Peggy to mix the three supplements together to make a palatable drink for Lisa.

For the next few hours Peggy, with Adam's help, alternated keeping Lisa's bandage moist and giving her the fortified vitamin drink. Lisa slept through the night, waking only briefly when Peggy and Bill took turns keeping the bandage soaked.

The next morning they removed the bandage and substituted vitamin E in ointment form rather than lotion, cream, or liquid. They had been taught that the ointment was the best to either prevent scarring or lessen the effects of scars, even on old scars.

Peggy asked her neighbor Emma, a registered nurse, to come over to examine Lisa's injury. When Emma arrived, Peggy told her the story, including how she had to pull the iron off Lisa's arm along with Lisa's burnt flesh. While the nurse was removing the bandage soaked in vitamin E, she scolded Peggy for not seeking professional help. However, upon examining Lisa's arm, Emma told Peggy that she had only one word to describe the wound: *amazing*. She said she had never seen such an immediate and effective healing process before. She added that the results Peggy had attained with the aloe vera plant and vitamin E could not have been attained with drugs. She then looked for any area of infection, but there was none to be found. Again, the nurse commented that what Peggy achieved with supplements alone was simply remarkable.

Perhaps Peggy should have gone to the hospital, but she didn't. Perhaps it was wrong for her to have practiced first aid herself, but she did. And now, so very many years later, Lisa recalls that morning and proudly shows that the burn from the iron left no scar.

Lisa was fortunate. Because of her mother's quick actions, she didn't have to suffer the effects of a serious burn. Perhaps you have seen or know about someone whose body has been scarred by a burn, including one caused by fire. The pain, both mental and physical, never seems to go away. But there still might be help for those suffering. According to Drs. Wilfred and Evan Shute, "It's never too late to use vitamin E in ointment form to lessen the effects of scarring, regardless of when it occurred."

I like telling this story. As a father, I'm proud of the way my daughter Peggy maintained her composure in a time of crisis. And, as a grandfather, I'm proud of the way my grandchildren, Lisa and Adam, responded to their mother's directives without hesitation.

21

SCARS - A KELOID

It was an exceptionally beautiful day in Santa Monica, California. A slight ocean breeze kept the temperature on the comfortable side in spite of the bright mid-afternoon sun. The people strolling along the boardwalk had dressed casually—most wearing shorts or bathing suits with cover-ups. After all, this was smack in the middle of the tourist season and, like most of my employees, I would rather be playing tourist than working. During my moment of wishing, a young mother and her son came strolling into the store. I guessed his age at about four years.

I did my usual cursory glance at the mother to establish if she had any noticeable deficiencies. Nothing visual with her; however, the little boy had a mark about the size of a silver dollar on the inside of his leg.

Curious, I said hello to him and knelt down and extended my hand for a high five. He smiled and responded accordingly. This gave me the opportunity to look at the mark on his leg. It wasn't a birthmark but a scar that had grown above the normal layer of skin. This type of scar is referred to as a keloid. His was about half an inch high and still looked painful, even though it had probably formed several months earlier.

I asked the mother what happened to cause the scarring.

She explained that her son got into the cabinet where she kept the cleaning products. The closed door was as secure as the childproof caps that only children can open, but it didn't keep him out of the cabinet and the bottle of lye. She added that it happened almost a year earlier when he had just turned three.

I asked her if she considered applying vitamin E to lessen the scarring.

She said that she and her husband had tried everything, including vitamin E, but that it hadn't had much of an effect.

I suggested that she had not used the right vitamin E.

She countered that she had used vitamin E lotion, then the cream, and finally the oil—all to no avail.

Again I said that she had not used the right vitamin E and showed her a bottle of vitamin E in ointment form. I then told her about Drs. Wilfred and Evan Shute, who wrote the book on vitamin E. Through extensive research and experimentation, they determined that vitamin E will reduce a scar, if not make it disappear altogether. They were referring, however, to the scarring that develops after a person suffers a survivable heart attack. Further studies determined that vitamin E has a similar effect on external scarring, but only if vitamin E is used in ointment form. The ointment adheres to the scar while the other forms are absorbed past the scar and into the body.

About two weeks later I received a phone called from a very excited young mother. She said they were amazed, as was their pediatrician, at the changes in the scar. It had decreased slightly in size, both in height and width. That was definitely a good sign, because keloids sometimes send out claw-like appenditures as they increase in size. This one, according to the doctor, had apparently stopped growing. The pain was gone, too. I received a second telephone call a few months later. The keloid was almost at the same level as the normal skin on his leg.

The mother also took my suggestion of giving her son a small amount of vitamin E internally. She did this by making a small hole in a 400-unit capsule and adding one drop to his glass of milk.

22

Scars - Prevention

I could readily see the open wounds on his face as he walked into the store. As he got closer I saw dried blood surrounding each of his wounds. He had countless stitches holding the wounds together, but they were red, oozing, and looked very painful. I greeted him and asked how I could help him.

"What can you do for my face so that I won't scar too much? I don't want to, in fact, I can't have any plastic surgery."

I did not ask him why, but guessed it might be for monetary reasons.

"Should I ask what happened?"

"I was in a bottle fight last Saturday night, and I guess you could say that I lost. I don't drink liquor, even beer, but a few of my friends and I got together, and, believe it or not, we were all drinking iced tea. Some guys from another table, who had been arguing among themselves, spilled some drink over one of my buddies. He commented that they should be a little more careful. That's all it took. Soon they were upon us with beer bottles that they had broken the bottom end off of. I held up a chair to protect myself, but someone threw a bottle that hit me across the side of my face." He pointed to one of the ugly gashes just below his eye. Several stitches were holding the skin together. "This one," he pointed to his forehead, "I got this one from a flying bottle. I don't know who threw it, but I caught it with my head. It took about ten stitches to close it up. But when it hit me I almost lost consciousness; that's when I got these." He pointed to the remainder of the wounds on his face and arm. "I can't fight, so I just tried to block their blows with the chair, but when I got hit in the head I dropped the chair, which left me an open target. Fortunately the police got there and arrested them before they killed any of us. I'm not sure what the D.A. is going to do about charges, but we have a lot of witnesses saying that they started the brawl. Anyway, my friends are much better off than me. So what can I do to keep them from scarring too much?"

I told him about the four-year-old boy whose scar had keloided, and how with the proper supplementation the scar eventually healed completely. I added that it did take time, of course, and that the little boy, still growing, was able to heal faster than an older person.

"I'll try anything." He bought some vitamin E oil and an ointment called hypericum. Unfortunately, vitamin E in an ointment form is no longer available, so he bought the hypericum to act as an ointment base. They mix well together, and hypericum is, according to the label, indicated for wounds. I saw this young man just two weeks later. I had to ask him if he was the same person who was in just recently, because his face no longer had open wounds.

"Yeah, I'm the one. Can you believe how my face is healing? I can't. Even the docs are amazed at my progress; in fact, they told my trainer that I could probably spar in a couple of months instead of the original prognosis of one year. I've told a couple of friends about that E stuff. I don't know how to thank you."

Trainer? Spar? Couldn't fight them? I asked, "Are you a professional fighter?"

"Yeah, sort of. Actually, I'm a professional kick boxer. If I weren't professional I could have, oh well, I didn't, but it turned out okay. Those guys are in jail where they belong and I'm healing up. So that's life. But hey, thanks for what you did. I really appreciate it."

He said he didn't live around here, but came in the first time because it was close to his bank. He also said it was lucky he had come into our store.

I'm glad I was able to tell him about the boy with the keloid and doubly glad he listened.

23

Scars
Can You Make Them Go Away?

How many times have you seen people, perhaps even in your own family, who have been burned and now carry horrible scars as a constant reminder? On many occasions I've seen such people and approached them with this story:

"I know of two doctors who have helped many people in your condition get relief from scarring and, in most cases, have the scars diminish to the point of disappearing. I'm selling you on an idea, not a product. What you do with it is up to you, but I pray that you will heed my advice. Your doctor might not agree, but these two doctors probably have more experience than yours with this therapy. Have no fear, because this product has but one side effect and it's a positive one. It will help your condition tremendously."

Then I would tell them how the two doctors used vitamin E internally and E ointment externally, and the mixing of E with hypericum ointment if E ointment is not available. By now they, or someone with them, would be writing down what I was saying. I'll never know whether or not they took my suggestion, as most of these encounters took place other than at my store or in my home town. Yes, I approached people everywhere and anywhere if I saw that they had a problem that could be corrected with nutritional supplements. That was my mission.

As you've already read, the two doctors I refer to in this story are the Drs. Wilfred and Evan Shute of Ontario, Canada. Their clinical work with vitamin E is outstanding, but is not accepted by many medical doctors. Their work included patients who had ulcerated amputation stubs; burns from explosions, fire, and hot steam; and children horribly burned by boiling water or open campfires. They used 600 units of vitamin E daily internally and vitamin E ointment topically, applied generously throughout the day and night. The results, according to them, were unbelievable.

Perhaps you, too, might consider relating this story to someone who has been disfigured or scarred.

Additionally, I have found that applying the vitamin E ointment on a post-surgical wound lessens the chance of internal scarring in the area of the surgery. For instance, there are times when, after back surgery, doctors have to "go back in" to remove scar tissue that has formed around the wound. After applying the E ointment mix, additional surgery to remove scar tissue was not needed. This treatment can be applied to any kind of surgery, including open heart, breast augmentation, or even to repair broken bones.

24

Depression
Something to Smile About

A smiling young woman of about twenty-five years of age entered my store late one afternoon. Because she was so nicely dressed, I assumed she was just coming home from work. I complimented her on the way she looked and asked what I could help her find. Without looking directly at me she said, jokingly, "A very rich, single man." And then added, "No, I'm just kidding. I'm looking for a multiple vitamin, something in a capsule form, because I just don't like swallowing tablets. And thank you for the compliment; that was very nice of you."

I directed her toward our multiple vitamin section and showed her a variety of encapsulated vitamins. I pointed out each of their attributes. She asked my opinion and eventually chose the one I suggested. Instead of paying and leaving, she joined me in a lengthy chat.

She told me about her moving to California, buying a home, finding a job, but, unfortunately, not finding a boyfriend. I was charmed by her continuous smile, which never waned throughout our conversation. She seemed to be so very happy with life, and I told her so.

She looked down at the floor and, in a sad tone, said, "But I'm not happy. It's a facade. In fact, I'm depressed. The anti-depressant the doctor gave me doesn't work. Sometimes I just want to stay home and cry. What do you have to make me truly happy? Do you sell a 'happy pill'?"

She was very attractive, had beautiful hair, walked and stood straight and tall, was well-dressed, was a good conversationalist, and had an unbelievable smile. What was causing her depression? Maybe it was internal; maybe it was caused by work, home life, or a past relationship. Could good nutrition help?

"Allow me to touch your hands, specifically, the palms of your hands. I want to see if they are moist."

"They're always moist. It's funny you should ask. How did you know?"

"Just a suspicion. Now I would like to ask you some questions."

Her answers indicated she was deficient in the mineral chromium. I gave her literature on low blood sugar and chromium, and the role they play in depression.

"Thank you, but I don't think a pill will help my problem."

Before I could ask what she meant, she continued, "Do you sell replacement faces?"

I was flabbergasted by her question. She was very attractive. Why would she ask about a replacement face?

"You're very attractive," I said almost apologetically.

"Thank you, except...all except for this. This ugly..." She looked up at me and then pointed at something on the right side of her face—something I had not noticed. She was no longer smiling.

I looked into her now-unsmiling eyes and said, "I would never have noticed that blemish if you hadn't stopped smiling."

My statement took her by surprise. She stepped back, looked at the floor and then back up at me with tears in her eyes. And then it happened. She was smiling once more—that beautiful infectious smile—and thanking me. As she completed her purchase, which included the mineral chromium, she smiled and laughed and then said goodbye.

To this day, I do not recall what it was she said she had, or what she pointed to. When she smiled it illuminated her entire face, and that was all I saw—her smile.

25

Phlebitis

As she grimaced with pain, she shoved her little son away from her, saying, "Don't do that to Mommy. I told you to stop it."

The four-year-old boy put his hands to his eyes and between tears whispered, "I'm sorry, Mommy."

She attempted to stoop down to his size but couldn't, so she called him over to her and held him against her left side, hugging him. She told him how sorry she was for pushing him and that she loved him very much.

"And I love you too, Mommy," was his reply.

This young boy had done what most small children do when they are excited, scared, or just in need of their mother's attention. They run to their mother and hug her. Because of the little guy's height, he had hugged her leg, her right leg. That's when the mother yelled with pain and pushed him away. He had obviously hurt her or hurt her already-injured leg.

"How bad is your injury?" I asked.

"Oh, he didn't injure me," she said, somewhat embarrassed when she realized I had witnessed the situation. "He was just giving his mommy some love." She smiled at her son and lightly patted him on the head.

"How bad is your injury?" I repeated the question.

The mother looked at me, annoyed that I persisted in questioning her.

"It's apparent that you're a first-time customer with us. Our customers know that I ask questions—lots of questions—as I'm doing with you. I realize that your son, by hugging you as he did, could not have caused you that much pain unless you were already in pain due to other circumstances. Did I guess correctly?"

"Yes. I have phlebitis, or thrombophlebitis as the doctor called it. It's in the area of my upper leg and exactly where my little guy hugged me."

"With that much pain, it would appear that it has become infected. How long have you been suffering with this?"

"Six weeks, and yes, it is infected. The doctor is considering surgery."

"Venous or arterial?"

She developed a quizzical look on her face. After a moment of thought, she answered, "It's in the vein; does that mean it's venous?"

"Yes, it does. Because of the extreme tenderness, I would also guess that it's a surface thrombus rather than a deep-veined condition."

The smile on her face meant she knew the answer to the question. "It's a surface thrombus. I was hit by a tennis racket—not on purpose—when my doubles partner swung her racket and hit my leg along with the tennis ball. I thought my leg would just be bruised, but the injury has developed into a full-blown infection."

"Thus you're probably on both antibiotics and anti-inflammatory drugs."

She nodded yes.

"I've never tried to talk a client out of taking their prescription drugs, and you are no exception. However, I have convinced a few clients to reconsider their impending operations. When are you due for surgery?"

"The doctor is doing more testing and is calling in a specialist who is a surgeon to examine me. That will be the end of next week." She saw me grimace after her last statement. "What?" she asked.

"What, what?" I countered.

"I saw the look on your face when I said I was to see a specialist. It's clear that you don't approve."

"If you were a surgeon whose income depended on doing surgery, would you be able to give an unbiased opinion?" I was sorry I had asked the question and told her so.

She accepted my apology. "I don't know what else to do. Do you have any suggestions? Do you think I shouldn't have the surgery, even if the specialist recommends it?" The stress in her voice was increasing.

"Mommy, are you okay? Are you going to cry because I hurt you?"

The young mother took a deep breath before telling her son that she was okay, that he didn't really hurt her that much, and, no, she wasn't going to cry.

"Look," I explained, "I got nosey and have created a mess. Again, I'm sorry. And, no, I'm not going to talk you out of surgery, because I don't know the severity of your problem. All I know is that you have severe pain, an infection, and are not improving. Until surgery occurs, you might consider taking vitamin C."

"Vitamin C for phlebitis?"

"Yes, and, based on the recommendations of Dr. Fred Klenner, in copious amounts."

"Copious. That sounds like a lot. Just how much is copious?"

"Dr. Klenner and others like him who believe in vitamin C usually prescribe upward of 5,000 milligrams taken at least six times a day." I could see her doing some quick math in her head. She finally responded.

"That's 30,000 milligrams. That's dangerous, isn't it?"

"Dangerous? According to them, no. You could be sensitive to that much vitamin C if you were to decide to take that quantity. 'Sensitive' meaning it could cause your stomach to rumble and you might develop loose bowels. If that were to happen, you would just decrease the amount until either of those conditions stopped. Extra calcium intake would also be indicated."

I could tell she was pondering what I had just said. "Would you excuse me while I make a telephone call?" she asked as she reached for her cell phone. "I need to call my husband for advice."

After a brief telephone conversation with her husband, she put the phone back into her purse and once again gave her son a little hug, saying, "Tommy, Mommy is going to be all better again. This man is going to help me." She turned to look at me and said, "Let's get started. My husband is decidedly against surgery and told me to purchase what I need, based on your suggestions or the suggestions of this Dr. Fred Klenner."

Together we reviewed the many articles written by this famous doctor, and, after one more telephone call to her husband, she decided to take what the doctor had recommended for his patients.

The surgery was never required, and within four weeks she was once again playing tennis, only this time without a doubles partner.

26

SMOKING

"Did you know that if you take vitamins A and C, you'll be able to smoke longer?" I asked the new customer who had said she was just looking.

"How can those vitamins make one live longer? I've never heard that before."

"These vitamins could lessen the chances of one getting lung cancer, or even the severity of it, thus, enabling you..."

She didn't let me finish, but interrupted me by saying, "That's cute. If I take them, I could live longer. Conversely, if I don't take them, it lessens my life expectancy. How did you know I smoke?"

Instead of answering her, I looked directly at her and took a deep breath.

"Oh, my gosh. You could smell it on me. It's that obvious, isn't it?"

"Yes, I could smell the smoke, but I could also tell by looking at your skin. Vitamin A, in particular, is a skin vitamin, and it appears, based on the texture of your skin, that you are deficient in this vitamin. Do your gums bleed when you brush your teeth?"

"Yes. Another deficiency of vitamin A?"

"That's a deficiency of vitamin C."

"What else are you finding wrong about me?"

"Well, what I first noticed about you is that you have a bandage on your arm. In fact, there is a slight bleeding as well. I'm guessing that it isn't a recent wound."

"No, it isn't. The doctor said I don't heal that well. I've had this sore for over three weeks, and it still bleeds when I barely hit or bump it. Is that also a deficiency of a vitamin?"

"Are you currently taking any vitamins?"

"Based on what you have been telling me, it should be rather apparent that I'm not."

"That's okay, you can start today. And I compliment you for considering taking vitamins—especially from me."

"I'm here because one of my co-workers suggested your place. Now I can understand why. You see things just as she said you did."

"Because you smoke, I see a need for vitamins A and C. But it's the non-healing of the sore that concerns me the most. That sore just increases the need for these vitamins because of the role they play as 'skin vitamins.' The healing of wounds depends on the formation of connective tissue, which cannot be synthesized without vitamin C. You probably get very little vitamin C, and your smoking uses up what you do get. Your wound will continue to break open and ultimately bleed unless you start increasing your intake of vitamin C in your diet."

"How much vitamin C?"

"The amount of vitamin C that you ingest is directly proportional to how fast you heal."

"And I need extra vitamin C because I smoke. That's relative as well, isn't it?"

"Yes."

"Okay, let's get started. Once I get well, is there something I could take that would lessen, no, stop me from smoking?"

I showed her an article that originated from the findings of Dr. Gershon Lesser. She said she was interested. After several weeks, she returned to my store. Her wound was now thoroughly healed, and she said she was anxious to start Dr. Lesser's program to stop smoking.The Doctor's regimen:

For two weeks take 2,000 mg of vitamin C and 50 mg of vitamin B-6 with each meal and at bedtime.

Take 500 mg of L-glutamine ½ hour before each meal and again at bedtime. Do not take with protein including milk.We had over a 50 percent success rate with this program and that's not taking into consideration those who didn't tell us their results. We assumed for them, it didn't work, but maybe it did, and they never got back to us.

27

VEGETARIANISM AND VITAMIN B-12

Occasionally, I struggle to find the slightest clue in determining someone's nutritional deficiency.

A girl of seventeen and her mother were visiting one of my stores to purchase some supplements. The girl was having severe digestive problems and wanted to purchase her usual supply of papaya enzymes, which, according to her mother, weren't working that well. Emily had tried various brands and enzyme formulas, even peppermint tea, with little or no results, and was currently using the papaya enzymes. Yes, she was under doctor's care, but he was unable to determine her problem in spite of extensive blood work and other kinds of testing. Hospitalization was becoming imminent.

At this point they decided to include me in discussions regarding Emily's problem. Her symptoms included poor digestion, tingling in the fingers, tiredness, and spots before her eyes.

When they told me these symptoms, especially the spots before the eyes, I thought I had found a solution. "Iron deficiency," I said. "You seem to be deficient in iron. What did the tests reveal about your iron count?"

"It was just a little low, so he put me on an iron supplement."

"Is it ferrous sulfate?"

Emily looked at her mother for the answer.

"Yes, it is ferrous sulfate."

"Emily, the doctor said your iron was just a little low, and yet the palms of your hands are pale, as is your face. Do you have excessive menstrual flow?"

Again she looked at her mother. I had obviously embarrassed her.

"Her periods are what the doctor referred to as 'scant.' He said that less is better than more, as more could mean a serious disease."

"Do you have bad breath?" I inquired.

"Yes, she does, but she won't admit to it. She brushes and flosses her teeth every time she eats, even while at school. But she still has that problem, although not all the time."

"Emily, let me see your tongue," I said.

She looked at her mother for support, who nodded that it was okay. Her tongue was coated, which could mean a deficiency of hydrochloric acid. This was unusual for anyone under thirty-five. I asked if they had considered this item.

"Yes, but I got awfully sick to my stomach. I told the doctor, and he said to stop it immediately."

I was stymied and told them so. I groped in my mind for an answer. There was something I had not thought to ask, something not tangible.

"Thank you, Bob, for trying. Emily and I have to go to the grocery store to buy something for dinner."

"What's for dinner?" I asked helplessly. I didn't want them to leave.

"I'm going to pick up a roast, beef roast. It's my husband's favorite."

"Emily, do you have a digestive problem when you eat beef?"

I still believed there was a question I had not asked, so I started with a question regarding hydrochloric acid.

"Oh, I don't eat meat. I'm a vegan" was her shocking answer—shocking because no one had mentioned it and I hadn't thought of asking it.

"You mean that you don't even eat animal crackers?" It was a fun question to ask vegetarians. It usually got a laugh, but this wasn't the case with Emily.

"No. I do not want my stomach to be a graveyard for little animals."

"Emily, how long have you been a vegan?"

"Are you going to try to talk me out of it, too? Mom and Dad tried, and so did the doctor, but I don't like eating meat. It makes me nauseous."

"Mom," I said to Emily's mother, "please give me a few more moments. I believe we might have the answer to this problem."

Again, Emily reiterated that she wasn't about to give up vegetarianism even if that was the cause of her distress.

"Emily, how long have you been a vegan? No, I'm not about to try to talk you out of being one, but I do need some answers."

"Almost four years."

"What kind of books did you study before practicing this kind of eating? I mean, did you read any books to enlighten you as to what foods you need to eat? Perhaps you read books about proper food combining, which teach you to be sure you get a complete protein at each meal. Did you read any books about being a vegan?"

"No. I just stopped eating meat, and then about six months later I stopped eating all dairy products and even eggs. I'm strictly a vegan, and I'm proud of it."

"What do you do to get vitamin B-12 in your diet?" I looked at her mother as I asked this question.

"The only B-12 I get is from the food I eat."

"Emily, vitamin B-12 is found in animal products—only in animals—not in vegetables." That was only a half-truth, as there are traces of B-12 in wheat germ and yeast. I didn't mention this to her, as I believed she would have said that she would include them in her diet. I felt that Emily was beyond any kind of food that would correct her current condition.

"Okay, Bob, what did the vegetarians do a hundred years ago? They didn't have a B-12 vitamin to take, and yet they survived. How do you explain that?"

"But Emily, they did eat meat, only they didn't know it."

"That's dumb. People know when they eat animals. It's not like eating a banana or some lettuce. See, you don't have an explanation."

"You and your mom were about to go to the grocery store. I presume that you would have bought your food at the same time—vegetables and an assortment of fruit."

She nodded in the affirmative.

"What's the first thing you do to your food when you get home and remove it from the grocery bag?"

"I either eat it or put it in the refrigerator."

"Don't you wash it before you eat it?"

"Of course I wash it. Doesn't everyone wash their food before eating it?"

"Do you suppose that hundreds of years ago the vegetarians washed their food before eating?"

"They didn't have to. Nobody used pesticides in those days."

"Emily, as I said earlier, and you just proved my point, vegetarians in those days did eat meat without knowing it. Allow me to explain. Let's say that one of them picked an apple off a tree. Do you suppose they peeled it before eating?"

"No, of course not." Emily seemed a little uncomfortable with my questioning.

"They just took a big bite out of this juicy red apple without peeling it. Right?"

"Yes, but what's the point?"

"When they ate the apple, they were also eating meat, without realizing it. Let me explain how and what I mean. Have you ever seen the eggs of a butterfly?"

"No."

"They are almost microscopic. You really have to look for them on, say, an apple. They are so tiny that one would probable pick an apple off a tree and just bite into it without seeing that they were eating the eggs of a butterfly, which was the meat they didn't realize they were getting. The source of their vitamin B-12. Emily, most nutrients are needed in what is called milligrams. Vitamin B-12 is measured in micrograms. It takes one thousand micrograms to equal one milligram and we only need about ten micrograms of B-12 a day. That's ten-thousandths of a milligram—not very much, yet attainable by eating the fruit off the trees or a vegetable from the ground. Emily, you have a glaring deficiency of vitamin B-12."

"Why didn't the doctor find out with all of the blood tests he's been doing?"

"Because you eat so many vegetables it wasn't that detectable. Vegetables provide much of the B vitamin called folic acid, and because of that, the blood appears normal. I should have realized it sooner. The combination of tiredness, tingling of the fingers, minimal bleeding during your menstrual cycle, and the poor digestion indicates a B-12 deficiency. Unfortunately, I didn't realize it until I asked your mom, "What's for dinner?"

Emily received injections of vitamin B-12 over the next few weeks and, by the time school started, was back to health. During this time, she began reading books about vegetarianism, learning how to compliment her food choices. She also included B-12 tablets in her diet.

28

Burning Feet

Doug—a big, strapping mechanic—entered my store early one afternoon and, in his booming, robust voice, asked, "Where's Bob?"

I heard him from the back room and walked to the front of the store. I noticed he was waving a piece of paper.

"Hi, Doug, what can I help you with?"

Still waving the paper he asked, "Burning feet. What vitamin am I lacking that will make my feet burn?" He started toward me, still waving the piece of paper.

"The same one I suggested you take for your allergies. Pantothenic acid."

"I'll be. The doctor was right. I just came from his office and decided to see you. I knew that you would know but I didn't expect the doctor to know. I'll be. He said I needed pantothenic acid and gave me this prescription. Can you fill it for me or do I have to go to the pharmacy?"

I looked at the prescription. It was for a very popular brand of an over-the-counter multiple vitamin. I said, "Doug, I have a bottle of this in the back room. I'll be right back." When I returned I handed him the bottle.

"Thanks, Bob," said Doug as he took the bottle from my hand. "Hey, wait a minute, this bottle is empty."

"Yes it is. Actually I just have it handy for when I give lectures. I can compare it with the brands I carry. Doug, check how much pantothenic acid is in this brand."

He started reading the label and said, "I don't see it listed. Does it have a different name or something?"

"It could be listed as pantothenic acid, calcium pantothenate, pantathine, or even vitamin B-5, but you won't find any of those names listed. The brand of vitamin the doctor prescribed does not contain any pantothenic acid."

Doug seemed stunned, and then his face started to turn red. It was obvious that he was getting angry. "I'll be. He told me my problem and then prescribed the wrong stuff. I'm glad I checked with you. What do you have for me that has pantothenic acid?"

"Doug, don't be too upset with the doctor. He diagnosed your condition correctly, and even though he didn't prescribe the correct vitamin, he did prescribe a vitamin instead of a drug. That in itself is an accomplishment. You can get this prescription for a multiple vitamin filled at the pharmacy and buy some supplemental B-5 from me."

"I'll get both of them here. Give me your best multiple and some extra pantothenic acid. If I had bought it from you when you suggested it for my allergies my feet probably wouldn't be burning."

"Perhaps, Doug, but now that you know that burning feet is another symptom, you probably realize how important it is for you to take it."

Burning feet is not an obvious symptom of a deficiency; however, when a deficiency of pantothenic acid seems apparent, I include the burning feet syndrome as one of the qualifying questions. I'm amazed how many *yes* answers I receive to my question about burning feet. Most people blame it on their shoes or standing on their feet for long periods of time. I remind them that pantothenic acid is the anti-stress vitamin, and that uncomfortable shoes or standing on one's feet for long periods could be considered stress. Stress is not just caused by a traumatic experience but could be triggered by the playing of loud music, the honking of a car horn, or even the crying of a baby or the barking of a dog. Pantothenic acid is used by the body in nerve transmissions and in the production of hormones that control our reactions to emotional and physical stress, including the fight-or-flight response.

29

Dizziness upon Arising

Trudy was a first-time customer. In fact, she wasn't a vitamin customer but was using my copying machine, which I used to make available to my current and potential customers. I should emphasize *potential* customers, because that was the primary purpose of putting the copying machine at the front of the store and then advertising on the front window that copies were available. I acquired many customers by just asking where they currently bought their vitamins. I always asked under the presumption that everyone took vitamins, even though that was far from true. Without knowing it, Trudy was about to become a vitamin customer. She had dropped one of her papers on the floor. After bending over to retrieve it, she got up very slowly.

"Bad back?" I asked. If I were to get a *yes* it would open the door for other questions, which eventually led to the person's purchasing a multitude of necessary supplements, especially a multiple mineral formula. With Trudy, I didn't get the usual *yes*.

She answered no. "I get very dizzy when getting up or standing up in a hurry, so I have to go rather slowly. I'm afraid I'll fall over or even faint."

"Are you seeing a doctor for this condition?" I always asked this question of new or potential customers.

"Yes, for about four months now, but it's not getting much better."

"What was the condition diagnosed as?"

"The doctor wasn't sure, but she thought it might be related to a yeast condition."

"Do you have a yeast condition?"

"No, I don't think so, but the doctor says I do. She says that sometimes the condition is dormant, so she is trying to activate it in order to treat it."

"A local medical doctor?"

"Yes, well, actually she is a pain specialist, but she said she could help me with these problems as well."

"Did you see her because of pain?"

"Yes, severe headaches. She said that these are all symptoms of my as-yet-undiscovered yeast infection."

"Migraine?"

"No, just headaches."

"What medicines has she prescribed for you?"

"Actually, she's not a medical doctor so she doesn't do any prescribing, but she's good. She has me on a whole bunch of different herbs. I didn't know that herbs are so expensive."

I proceeded to ask Trudy several questions relating to pantothenic acid deficiency. She answered yes to almost all of them. "Based on your answers, it appears that you are deficient in pantothenic acid."

"What's that?"

"It is vitamin B-5 but is usually referred to by its longer name, pantothenic acid. Many of your symptoms could be corrected by adding this vitamin to your diet. It is even indicated for yeast infections by many nutritional doctors."

"Even the dizziness? This could be caused by a lack of this vitamin?"

"Most definitely."

"How long do I have to take this vitamin before I see results?"

"If the dizziness is due to a deficiency, you should see results in two weeks or less."

Trudy's dizziness was relieved in less than four days. Except for a few minor incidents, her headaches were relieved in one day. Most of her other symptoms disappeared in about a month. She also convinced three other patients of the "pain doctor" to take our Body Language Questionnaire and they, too, became regular customers. Trudy confided that she was spending over $75 a week on herbs and was upset that her condition was corrected for less than $10.

I reminded Trudy that all stress, including that which she was displaying for the doctor, affects the body in a negative way. It's better to get the negatives out of one's life.

At one of the many lectures I have attended, it was explained that the adrenal glands compensate for the slightest change in elevation, even the getting up from a lying or sitting position. This condition is called postural hypotension.

30

Dizziness - Try Coughing

Many years ago I was counseling a mother and her two teenage children. Because an employee was using the seating area, we decided to sit on the floor, which had just been cleaned that morning. After the counseling session was over, I got up and offered my hand to the mother.

"Oh, no, Bob. Thanks, but I have to get up very slowly. So does my daughter. We both get very dizzy if we get up too fast."

"Maybe we should all stay seated and discuss the two of you—nutritionally I mean."

"Not today, but next week for sure. We have to meet my sister and her family for lunch." The daughter was trying to get up on one knee, but the mother was still in a sitting position on the floor.

"Try coughing," I said to the daughter.

"What?"

"Try coughing. A deep cough, one that's coming from the chest. Do it two or three times, and then you'll be able to get up without being dizzy."

The mother and daughter looked at each other. Who was going to do it first? After some encouragement from the son, his sister coughed twice and started to get up.

"Not a deep enough cough. It must come from the chest, not the throat," I said and then gave them an example. The daughter followed my instructions and started to get up once again—first on one knee and then the other.

"Mom, no dizziness. At least not yet." As she started to rise once again she suddenly stopped and said that she got a little dizzy and then, without my telling her to do so, coughed once again. This time she was able to stand without any dizziness whatsoever.

"Mom!" she exclaimed, "I did it! It really worked! Now you try it."

Her mother opted not to try coughing and, after several minutes, was able to get up with the help of her children. She did call me the next day to say that, with her husband at her side, she got up from a sitting position without the usual dizziness, all because of coughing.

After a few days of taking pantothenic acid, both the mother and daughter reported that their dizziness occurred only rarely. That's when they were convinced they needed to include the supplement in their diet.

Many years earlier I, too, would get dizzy when arising from a sitting position. I reasoned that if I coughed I would be forcing blood into my brain and thus alleviate the lack of blood, which I believed caused the dizziness to occur. After a certain amount of experimentation, coughing before arising allowed me to change positions without dizziness. Eventually I discovered pantothenic acid, and since taking the supplement I have never been bothered with dizziness again. I have often wondered if deep coughing would correct or lessen the effects of a heart attack. Just recently, I read an article by Dr. Kurt Donsbach reporting that coughing could save a person's life if he or she were having a heart attack. He stated that the coughing promoted the flow of blood into the heart.

31

Adrenal Insufficiency

Whenever anyone wore sunglasses while shopping at my store, I got curious. Of course it could be a convenience factor; it's easier to leave them on than to take them off and find a place to put them. But any time I saw someone wearing sunglasses indoors I looked for clues to noticeable nutrient deficiencies. Was his or her hair dry? Did the person's fingernails appear brittle or was she wearing acrylics? Did he or she have a stuffy nose?

This particular young lady didn't have any of these conditions, but there were two others that caused me to ask her if she had headaches or allergies. She answered yes to both.

"How did you know?" she asked.

I lied and told her it was a guess.

Then she took off her sunglasses, confirming my suspicion. Possible adrenal gland problem.

The first clue was an extreme amount of facial hair, especially around the mouth and temple. The second was the contour of her body. When she took her glasses off, I saw the third. Dark circles under her eyes indicated adrenal problems. Yes, any of these conditions could have been caused by a myriad of things, but I suspected adrenal dysfunction. I asked her about headaches and allergies to confirm my intimations. I received a multitude of *yeses*, so many that I suggested she make an appointment with her doctor, although I did feel comfortable selling her pantothenic acid. She called me a few weeks later saying that the doctor had indeed diagnosed her as having a minor problem with her adrenal cortex. After telling him how it had helped her tremendously with her headaches, allergies, and dizziness, the doctor advised her to continue with the pantothenic acid.

32

Carpal Tunnel Syndrome - Men

This problem is not just limited to women, nor does it affect those who are not strong. Big Dale is strong and has a great, bellowing voice. As he entered my store one fine day, he greeted me with his rousing "Hello" and then extended his left hand, twisting it to shake my right hand. His right hand was encased in bandages, which, of course, caused me to ask, "What's the matter with the arm?"

"Oh, I've got what they call carpal tunnel syndrome. In fact, I have it in both arms, but they could only do surgery on one arm at a time. It doesn't hurt much, but it's an inconvenience that's costing my wife and me a lot of income. I'm not looking forward to three more weeks with the bandage on this arm and then two months on the left arm." He made a wry face and continued, "The doc says it was caused by being a mechanic. I guess I do too much twisting and turning when I'm using my tools."

"Dale, you are a rarity," I exclaimed.

"Why?"

"Carpal tunnel syndrome affects women more than men. It's also more common among those who are pregnant, going through menopause, or taking oral contraceptives. Now, if a person is on hemodialysis for his or her kidneys, and that includes men as well as women, then he or she too is prone to carpal tunnel syndrome."

"Why?" he asked again.

"It has been determined that these people tend to be deficient in vitamin B-6."

"Should I be taking B-6 then, and, if so, why didn't the doctor prescribe it?"

"Dale, being out of work is one thing, and the cost of medical bills adds up rather quickly, too. First, let's talk about improving your healing process so you won't be suffering so long, both financially and physically. Then we can talk about B-6."

We discussed the reasons for taking his multiple vitamin at least two times a day instead of just once. Unfortunately, in Dale's case, his "once" meant "once in awhile." An extra supply of the B vitamins plays an integral part not only in the healing process but also in combating the stress that any injury places on the body. I suggested that Dale include extra vitamin C, bromelain, and pantothenic acid in his healing regimen. To preclude any prostate problems, he was already taking vitamin E and some zinc his doctor had recommended. I then sold him a multiple mineral complex, advising him that single supplements, such as zinc, taken over a prolonged period of time could upset the balance of the rest of the nutrients.

Because Dale was very receptive to my suggestions, I decided that now was the right time to test the depth of his confidence in me. I said, "Dale, thank you for the trust you've shown me. Could you stretch that trust enough to try an experiment over the next few weeks while your right arm is in the process of healing?"

There wasn't the slightest hesitation in his response. Of course he agreed. He appreciated the successes we had had just in the past year alone in correcting conditions his wife and his mother had developed through nutrient deficiencies. "Bob, let's not forget that I'm on your side of the fence. What can I do to help?" he asked.

"Dale, it's about the vitamin B-6 your doctor didn't prescribe. Maybe he's not aware of the many studies advocating this vitamin. Or maybe he read a study that concluded it doesn't work that well for carpal tunnel. I believe that any negative studies are because of the duration required for results. People don't like taking a pill once a day, let alone four times a day, as is required for B-6 therapy. And again, it takes up to three months before results are produced. People become impatient."

"Bob, there's one thing about you, you're always honest with people. That's why, if it's affordable, I'll go along with whatever you suggest."

"You'll have to be consistent in taking your multiple vitamin at least two times a day. It's to ensure that you're getting adequate amounts of vitamin B-2, as this compliments the extra B-6. You can determine your multiple vitamin needs by checking the color of your urine. It should be a bright yellow throughout the day, and, if it isn't, you'll need to increase taking your multivitamin accordingly."

"Is it the multivitamin that causes the bright yellow color?" he asked.

"Actually, Dale, it's the vitamin B-2. Many people believe vitamin C causes the yellow color, but it's the B-2."

He bought a bottle of vitamin B-6 in the 25 mg strength and promised to take one pill with each meal and another at bedtime. I reminded him again that he must continue taking his multivitamin as well. I also told him that B-6 is a diuretic and that he should be prepared to visit the bathroom a lot. He laughed and gave me a big bear hug goodbye.

I saw Big Dale about two months later. The doctor had removed the bandages from his right arm, revealing an ugly scar. The arm was still sore from the operation and there was still residual pain in his wrist. I told him about using arnica montana, both topically and orally, and that it is effective in relieving this kind of pain. I also insisted he tell his doctor all the nutrients he was taking.

He looked at me and said in a somewhat growling tone, "Are you kidding? He only knows about cutting and poisoning through his operations and drugs. Look at what he did to me." Dale showed me his scar again. I assured him that it was only temporary and that there was a combination of supplements to lessen the scaring. (See Story 23).

I then asked him about his left arm, and his answer was an unprintable profanity. He said his left arm tingled but was no longer painful, and that was only when he twisted or turned it while at work. He said he was sorry he had had the operation, not only because it didn't totally make him well, but also because of all the pain and misery he had suffered and the work and income he had lost. If there was ever a true convert to the health industry, Dale was the epitome. I told him about including some stretching exercises that would lessen the need for surgery even more

Months later, Big Dale would sometimes complain of aches in his right arm, but his left arm never bothered him again.

Let's see: the cost of the operation, many visits to the doctor, medication, a short hospital stay, loss of work, loss of income, and sitting and being an invalid for that length of time versus the cost of two bottles of vitamin B-6. Hmmm, it certainly seems worth trying before surgery. If surgery is necessary, bromelain should be incorporated into the diet. One should start this regimen at least three or four days prior to surgery and, for maximum benefit, continue after surgery for a minimum of two to three weeks.

33

Carpal Tunnel Syndrome - Women

One evening my wife, Pat, asked me to bring home a loaf of bread after work. Vivian was the cashier working the express lane that night. She told me they had put her in this checkstand because she couldn't lift many things and especially not anything heavy. She then showed me her arms, which were encased in leather-like braces.

"Carpal tunnel syndrome?" I asked.

"Why yes, how did you know? Oh, that was a dumb question. You're the guy who looks at people and sees deficiencies. Hi, Bob, I didn't recognize you right away. Hey, tell me, Bob, what deficiencies could cause these?" She raised both arms to show off her twin braces. "There seems to be an epidemic at this store. Seems like everyone here has this problem."

"Do you all go to the same doctor?" I asked.

"Yes, how did you know? He's our workman's comp. doctor. He's good. I mean, who knew what carpal tunnel syndrome was except him?"

"And does he do the surgery as well?" I asked.

"Surgery? He has never mentioned that I might need surgery. Anyway, he's not a surgeon, just a regular doctor. You know, a Dr. Welby type."

"Vivian, do you have the usual premenstrual problems, like bloating, swelling, and tenderness?" I asked. I realize that this question could be very embarrassing to many people, but Vivian was a regular customer of ours, and although I have not waited on her personally, my employees have helped with her children's problems. Additionally, there were no other customers in her line who could have overheard my question.

"Why yes, doesn't every woman?" she countered.

"No, not every woman. Particularly, our customers who have confided in us about this problem. Vivian, perhaps we can correct two problems at once. No, three. Both of your arms as well as your premenstrual witchiness."

"Who said I was witchy?" she asked with a huge grin. Then she asked, "Do you mean you can correct that as well?"

"Probably," I answered.

"Four!" she exclaimed. "You're going to correct four of my problems. What do I need to do, or take?"

The next day, Vivian started her B-6 therapy rather enthusiastically. Her menstrual cycle was to start within the next two days, so she was rather eager to get the experiment started. A week later, I again needed to pick up a few grocery items on my way home from work. I made it a point to go through Vivian's line.

"Hey, Vivian, what happened to your fashionable braces?"

"Don't need them anymore. And thanks to you, I am a lovable, sweet, no-longer-bloated, and cured lady. All in a week's time. Will this good feeling continue or will I be faced with these problems next month? Am I cured?"

"Vivian, now you know how to correct these problems, so if they come back start the B-6 regimen again, but only take it during that time of the month."

"Sounds too simple."

"It doesn't have to be complicated to work."

Several of Vivian's co-workers came in to buy B-6 for their problem—no, two problems.

34

Capillary Fragility

Most everyone is familiar with what a vein or an artery is, but how many people know what venules or arterioles are? And what is a capillary? Venules, arterioles, and capillaries form a vast network of blood vessels that includes the arteries, veins, and heart. Collectively, these components make up the cardiovascular system, which delivers fresh, oxygenated blood from the heart to all parts of the body. The heart pumps this nutrient-filled blood through the arteries down to smaller arteries called arterioles. The arterioles transport this fresh blood to the capillaries, where the cells of the body receive the oxygen, nutrients, hormones, and antibodies and also where the wastes are collected. Upon completion of the work of the capillaries, the used blood enters the venules and then moves into the veins for its return to the heart for re-oxygenation. It's for the functioning of the capillaries, these tiniest of blood vessels, that the entire cardiovascular system exists.

The entire circulatory system, from the arteries to the arterioles, venules, and the veins, is impermeable—watertight or blood-tight. Even the tiniest of blood cells are unable to permeate through these impenetrable walls—except for the capillaries, which must be permeable. They must be able to allow the nutrient-rich fluid from the bloodstream to seep out of this divergent system and merge with the fluid that surrounds all the body's cells. Then this fluid must be able to seep back into the capillaries.

For this seepage and reverse seepage to come about, the walls of the capillaries must be permeable, but not too permeable. When the capillaries are too fragile and break—or too permeable—blood accumulates, causing the appearance of bruise marks on the skin. When skin bruises easily it indicates that the capillaries are too breakable. Diet, prescription drugs, smoking, and various illnesses, including hypothyroidism, cause brittle capillaries.

Many studies have established that vitamin C and bioflavonoids decrease capillary fragility and help prevent abnormal permeability. And yet bioflavonoids, originally called vitamin P or the "non-vitamin," are considered by the U.S. Food and Drug Administration (FDA) to have little or no nutritional value.

Many stories in this book describe the use of bioflavonoids and their effectiveness in treating the associated maladies.

35

Bruises

It looked as if his blood was seeping through his skin. That was my first experience seeing capillary fragility, a condition whereby blood accumulates in the skin and has the appearance of bruise marks. No doubt you've seen those purple bruise marks yourself, especially in older people. The medical profession says that fragile capillaries are an inevitable malady for people in their seventies or eighties. Walt, however, was only in his late forties.

Walt was the state manager for a life insurance company I had applied to work with on a part-time basis. I enrolled in their training classes, read their many manuals, and took several exams. I scored so high on the company's final test that Paul, my manager, said I was to work solely with Walt instead of with him and the other recruits. I was flattered. Walt was to be my personal mentor in preparing for the California State test, and I was to begin working with him that particular afternoon.

Later that day, Paul introduced me to Walt. He had a slight build, a beautiful head of white hair, a very friendly smile, and, I would guess, was at least sixty-five years old. His face was very pale. After our introduction, Walt and I went into Paul's office for privacy to map out my training schedule. When he removed his suit coat, I noticed the many purple marks on his hands and arms. They were visible even through the long sleeves of his white dress shirt. This was my first close-up experience with the condition medically called "capillary fragility," or capillaries that are so fragile they break easily.

That was when I learned that I was a poor judge of age.

"These purple marks," said Walt, "usually occur in older people. The doctors call it "thin skin," and they say it's part of growing old. One of my doctors said it's caused by exposure to the sun. In my case, the blood thinners and cortisone that were prescribed for my heart cause these marks. Bob, don't let this gray hair fool you, I'm only forty-seven years old. The gray was also caused by my medication."

His eyes were no longer blue but had a grayish color. The whites of his eyes were filled with blood—not the usual red lines people have, but big blotches of blood. I couldn't help hurting for my new friend.

"It's okay, Bob. I'm under the best of the best doctors' care in the state. I can only hope and pray that they know what they're doing."

We ended the conversation and began a two-hour session to determine the course we would follow in his teaching me about life insurance. It was concluded that we would begin our tandem teaching and learning on the following Monday evening.

It was Friday.

Early Monday morning I received a call from Paul. He informed me that Walt had died Sunday night. He had literally bled to death through his skin. My first reaction was shock. Then I got angry. Angry at his doctors for allowing this tragedy to happen. After awhile the anger dissipated and was replaced by sorrow. Sorrow for Walt and his family.

Perhaps his dying was part of my destiny. I didn't continue selling insurance, and, after several years, I entered the field of nutrition. That was when

I learned about bioflavonoids. If only I had known about them when I met Walt. If only the doctors had considered bioflavonoids as part of their therapy for him. If, if, if...

36

BIOFLAVONOIDS

When I bought some plants for the store I noticed that the cashier, a woman in her late sixties, had bruise marks around her wrist. I asked what she was doing to correct this condition.

"The doctor said it's thin skin and there is no cure. Anyway, I shouldn't be wearing my bracelets; that only makes the bruising worse."

I suggested a bioflavonoid regimen. Several weeks later, I went to the same nursery to buy some fertilizer for the plants. The same cashier checked out my purchase and then recognized me. "You're the guy who told me about bioflavonoids. Look. No more bruising. Now I can wear my bracelets again."

It was obvious that the supplement had brought the joy of wearing bracelets into her life again. What a great testimonial for bioflavonoids and another blow to the medical theory that there is no cure.

Another story...

My wife, Pat, and I would trade off each morning as to who would walk the two blocks to the post office. This morning it was my turn, and I wanted to be there before the crowd. It was 8:00 a.m. as I entered through the front door to retrieve the mail from my box. I could not help noticing a young woman standing at one of the vacated counters. She was wearing shorts and a halter-top, and was barefoot. She was probably the driver of the mini-van parked outside that was loaded with children and beach toys. Yes, I noticed her legs—but I always look at people—and it was obvious to me that she bruised easily. There is a particular texture to skin that tells me a person bruises easily, like a blotching or vein-like lines, which are most apparent on the upper arms and the legs. If you bruise easily, compare your skin to someone who does not bruise to see if you can distinguish the different nature of the skin.

I was in a dilemma. Eight o'clock in the morning, just the two of us, and she's dressed as she is. I argued in my mind as to whether or not I should say something. I picked up my mail from the P.O. box and, at another counter, separated the mail orders from the bills. Yes, I could have done this chore at the store, but I was still deliberating what to do. I decided to leave and not say anything. As I got to the door, I stopped, did an about-face, and walked back to the counter. I reached into the trash and retrieved one of the envelopes I had just discarded. I wrote:

For bruise marks:

Take one bioflavonoid capsule three times a day. Within two weeks, your bruising will lessen considerably. Take one capsule a day thereafter until bruising disappears.

Upon completion of the note, I walked over to the woman and handed her the envelope and said, "Here, this is yours."

This was something I never did at my store, write down how a vitamin should be taken. Because of the circumstances, I did what I believed needed to be done.

Did she ever read the note? I don't know. If she did, would she buy and try the bioflavonoids? Probably not, especially if she first discussed it with her doctor. I know that sounds rather cynical toward doctors, but read the next story and you'll understand why I feel this way.

37

Bioflavonoids and the Lost Lease

My wife, Pat, and I had had our first store for three months when two pharmacists approached me. They wanted me to open a vitamin section in their pharmacy. Since it was an opportunity to expand our sales, we agreed, and I signed a three-year lease with them.

Their pharmacy catered mostly to a clientele over sixty. Most every one of them bruised. I was in my heyday.

"Good morning," I would say, "what is the doctor doing for your bruise marks?"

Most often the answer would be, "I have thin skin. There's nothing that can be done."

The majority of the time I sold them bioflavonoids, which they bought happily. I had several successful months at the pharmacy and was extremely pleased with the increase in sales. Late one evening, I received a call from my pharmacist landlords. They had to see me the next morning before seven o'clock.

"Bob," they said almost in unison. "Bob, we have to terminate your lease."

I was dumbfounded.

They continued. "We have had many, many complaints from our doctor clientele that you are embarrassing them with their patients. They had told their patients that bruise marks are a part of growing older and cannot be cured, and your bioflavonoid supplement is curing their patients' problems. The doctors gave us an ultimatum: If you don't stop telling their patients about bioflavonoids, they will suggest to their patients that they have their prescriptions filled elsewhere."

I was being asked to break my lease with no penalties, a full refund of my deposits, and to just leave. Never mind the patients. Never mind how the addition of one nutrient corrected a condition that changed the attitude of these elderly people. Of course, I chose to leave the mentality of my landlords. I could only imagine what their next reason for my leaving would be.

I packed up my vitamins, and as I was leaving the pharmacy for the last time, one elderly customer hugged me goodbye and said, "Now we don't have anybody here to trust anymore."

38

Motion Sickness

I absolutely never take vitamin B-6 with me when I go fishing; I don't get seasick. But on one fishing trip I made an exception. Devin, a dear friend and fishing buddy, asked me to go ocean fishing with him and one of his co-workers. I knew that Devin was a hardy soul who wasn't affected by the ocean waves, but I didn't know about his buddy. In spite of Devin's assurance I packed some B-6 and a lemon, just in case. His buddy cancelled the evening before; however, another of Devin's co-workers asked if she could go in his stead. No, she had never been in a small, 16-foot fishing boat before, not even on a lake.

This is sort of a "good news, bad news" story. Yes, the three of us took off in that rowboat. The weather was beautiful, and the fishing turned out to be better than expected. In fact, Devin caught a sleek barracuda that measured in excess of twenty-six inches.

Perhaps it was the blood from the fish, maybe the jostling in this small boat, or just the slight rolling of the water—Devin's friend got sick—really sick. Selfishly, all I could think was, "There goes my fishing trip." Then I remembered the vitamin B-6.

I had both read and heard stories about the helpfulness of this vitamin in preventing and correcting motion sickness of any kind, but this was my first experience with it. "Here, take this." It was more of a demand on my part.

"What is it?" she asked between her episodes of feeding the fish.

"Just take it," Devin said without knowing what I was offering her. "It'll help you get better." He looked at me for assurance.

I nodded yes.

She took the B-6. Fortunately, it stayed down long enough to be effective. Between the B-6 and sucking on the slices of lemon, our little sailor felt better in half an hour's time. She wanted to fish some more.

On the way home from this most memorable day, I discussed other symptoms of vitamin B-6 deficiency with Devin's friend. When I learned that she suffered from severe premenstrual symptoms, I gave her the bottle of B-6 and suggested she consider taking it. Devin told me later that she took my advice and never needed to miss work again due to PMS.

After that, when anyone mentioned that he or she was going fishing, boating, riding in a car, flying, or going to an amusement park, I would suggest including vitamin B-6 for those who are prone to motion sickness. It works!

39

Pregnancy and Nausea

A young couple held hands as they entered my store, both smiling, both seeming very happy. The woman stopped suddenly, gasped, and jerked her hand out of his to cover her mouth. This made her voice sound garbled as she said, "Honey, I've got to leave, right now!"

At the same time, she bolted toward the front door of my store, taking a small plastic bag out of her pocket and putting it up to her face. Morning sickness, I guessed, the scourge of pregnant women.

"She can't go anywhere without her baggie," her husband said. "The doctor told us that she has one of the worst cases he's ever seen. He called it 'spontaneous disgorge.' We just call it plain old mid-morning sickness, except it happens all the time. My poor little wifey."

"I'll get her a glass of water."

"Thank you, that's very considerate, but not too much. She can't even hold water down. Her vomiting's that bad."

The wife returned and apologized for having her attack. I noticed she had a new baggie grasped firmly in her hand. She took the glass in her empty hand, but hesitated before taking a drink. Was she thinking it might make her vomit again? Slowly and very deliberately, she took a sip of the water and then hesitated. At first she seemed to allow the liquid to languish on her tongue before swallowing it. Then, the look on her face, her pale face, seemed to say that the water seemed fine in her stomach. She sipped at the water again.

"What trimester of pregnancy are you in?" I asked, expecting her to say it was her first.

"I'm starting my third trimester next week, and thank you for the water."

"You're welcome for the water, but I can't believe that after six months you're still having morning sickness."

"Yes. I didn't think it's supposed to last this long. I feel so weak."

Silently I agreed with her. Poor little mother-to-be. Her pregnancy did not have to be so traumatic.

"It's debilitating," her husband said. Then he asked, "Is there anything you can suggest for the nausea? We were told that you could help us."

"Sir, as much as I would like to help, I am unable to."

"Why, aren't you the one who helps people who are hurting? That's why we came to see you." He was pleading now.

"I'm not able to, especially because your wife is pregnant. The severity and duration of her morning sickness, her feeling of weakness, and her already being under doctor's care—I really can't get involved with this situation. I truly am sorry, and I hurt for you both."

"Any suggestions at all?" the wife urged.

"Ask your doctor if he'll give you an injection of vitamin B-6. And he should check you for potassium—you could be very low because of the continuous vomiting." For emphasis I added, "Your feeling of weakness could be caused by many things, most probably by a deficiency of potassium."

This was all I could do. Hopefully, their doctor would consider my suggestions.

They thanked me and, as they walked out of my store, again holding hands, I said a silent prayer for them. The following Thursday the husband came back to tell me what had happened. Absolutely nothing. They had told their doctor what I recommended. The doctor asked if they wanted him to continue being their obstetrician, "Or do you want that vitamin salesman to be your doctor? Ask him how much medical training he has to make such rash suggestions."

"Bob, we're desperate. Lynne is supposed to be the matron of honor for her sister's wedding this Saturday. That's the day after tomorrow! How can she walk down the aisle with a bouquet in one hand and a baggie in the other? And what would she do if she got sick in the middle of the vows? This seems hopeless."

No, because I didn't practice medicine I couldn't get personally involved in this situation, but I knew of someone who could get involved. "Excuse me a moment," I said to the frustrated husband. I walked over to my business card file, found the right card, dialed the number, and waited for someone to answer.

"Doctor's office."

"Good afternoon. This is Bob at the vitamin store. Is the doctor able to see someone at this time? It's not an emergency in the usual sense, but it is to the people I'm sending over."

"Sure, Bob, send them over," said the caring voice of the receptionist. "They might have to wait, but only for a short while. I'll squeeze them in as quickly as possible."

How professional and yet understanding. I don't usually interfere with a doctor and his patient, but the severity of this situation required more than the usual help. This woman should not have had the depth and duration of morning sickness she had been suffering. And now it threatened an entire wedding party. So I got involved more than usual. As I handed the business card to the husband, I couldn't help seeing the tears swell in his eyes.

He looked at the card, looked up at me, and, without saying a word, gave me a big hug. He started toward the front door but stopped, turned around, and said, "They were right! I knew you could help us!" and hurried to his wife, who was waiting in the car.

About four hours later, I received a call from the husband. They had fired their original doctor and gone with the one I recommended. The new doctor gave the pregnant wife an injection of vitamin B-6 and a prescription for potassium. Recognizing that this young mother-to-be was in dire need of them, the doctor prescribed these two supplements. It was not at my suggestion. Yes, two days later she was able to perform her duties as matron of honor without getting nauseated. In fact, after the initial injection of vitamin B-6 she never had another episode of vomiting. The wedding went well, as did the rest of the pregnancy.

40

Emphysema

How many times have you heard the labored breathing of someone suffering from emphysema? Perhaps a friend or a relative or even a co-worker has this affliction. Many blame this disease on smoking, or on secondary smoke, or even on the increase of smog in our cities. It is almost impossible to treat, and yet I had the experience of lessening the effect of this disease on one person in particular.

I was on a fishing trip with one of my dearest friends. Prior to fishing, Dick and I were having breakfast. We were sitting at the breakfast bar in a little town called Searchlight, Nevada, adjacent to the mighty Colorado River. The guy next to us was nursing his coffee and small-talking with the waitress. His breathing was extremely difficult, as if he was fighting for enough air to catch his next breath. I made no comment, at least not right then. Dick and I were enjoying our breakfast in spite of his noisy breathing.

"Bob, look at that couple over there next to the coat rack," exclaimed Dick.

I looked in the suggested direction and saw the couple Dick was referring to. They were having breakfast, too.

"So?" I asked.

"Look, he's eating and she's smoking!" he exclaimed.

Again I answered, "So?"

"Look at the tubes in his nose. He can't breathe, and she's blowing smoke in his face!"

The guy had a tube in each nostril with the other ends leading to an oxygen tank, which was sitting on a two-wheel cart next to his chair. Dick was thoroughly disgusted with what he saw.

"How stupid that woman is. He can't breathe, needs oxygen, and she won't stop smoking! She could blow the place up if she gets any more careless." He added, "She is one of the most callous and uncaring women I've ever seen! It makes me sick." With that Dick turned away and set his fork down. "With life as precious and limited as it is, she's taking away minutes or even hours from him just because of her smoking habit. She disgusts me, Bob, I've got to say something to her."

"Dick, before you go over, look at the guy's shirt pocket."

Dick let out a profanity and said, "I can't believe it. He has his own pack of cigarettes in his pocket. Now I don't feel sorry for them. They're both stupid."

The guy next to us chimed in, "Hey, buddy, he's got what I've got, emphysema. There's no cure, so why not let them live and die in peace? They're friends of everybody in here. We've all tried to tell them to stop, but they don't listen. Heavy smoking caused their problem. I think they said they smoked over three packs a day for more than fifty years."

The waitress nodded in agreement and then added, "Ben never did smoke. He got his emphysema from living in L.A., with all of that smog."

"And the paint fumes too, I guess. I was a painter all my life," said Ben.

Now it was my turn. "Ben, let's talk."

Ben became a mail order customer of ours and continued buying from us for many years. During the time he did buy from us he "got almost cured," as he would say. He wasn't cured, but he did improve tremendously. His problem was that he needed oxygen, and vitamin E provides oxygen in generous amounts.

Because of the recommended dosage of Drs. Wilbert and Evan Shute, Ben decided that 800 units was not enough, so he doubled the amount and then increased the original amount again by half. He leveled off at 2,000 units a day, and his breathing became less labored. Now it was time to improve the connective tissue of his lungs, and that required other supplements. The Body Language Questionnaire showed that Ben was seriously deficient in vitamins A and C, as well as folic acid. He started a regimen high in these supplements.

He also changed his eating habits in order to get more protein, which helped improve his immune system.

Within a few months, Ben was able to take walks for a mile or more a day. He always longed to walk the desert country of Nevada and watch the ever-changing landscape. His mail orders for more product always included a progress report, so that we could know how he was doing.

What about the other couple at that breakfast bar, the smokers? We learned that they passed away during the three years Ben was our customer. And after three years of watching Ben's progress, we never did find out what happened to him. One day, without explanation, his orders stopped, and we never heard from him again. We are comforted by the fact that at least he made a clear improvement in his life and lifestyle during the time we knew him.

41

Asthma

I've seen people grimace with pain as the limited amount of oxygen they breathe in finally reaches their lungs. But seeing a child struggling to take a deep breath, or even trying to breathe normally, hurts me almost as deeply as it hurts them.

Sandy, a local newspaper salesperson, came into my store early one afternoon to bring me an ad copy I needed to proofread before publishing. She had two little children with her.

"Hi, Bob. I apologize for having to bring my children with me, I know it's unprofessional, but I had to pick them up earlier than usual from school."

Sandy was a very aggressive salesperson for whom I had a lot of respect. I knew she was a divorced mother with two children, but I had not realized how young they were until seeing them that day.

"Don't kid me, Sandy, you brought them with you to show them off," I said with a grin. "And they are beautiful children. My compliments to you."

"Thank you. Yes, I think they are beautiful too. Bob, here's your ad copy. Proofread it and call me tomorrow if there are any corrections or additions. Excuse me for hurrying, but I want to get home as soon as possible."

I could have just said "thank you" and "goodbye" to Sandy and her children, but I noticed something I needed to ask her about.

"Sandy, does your daughter always breathe through her mouth?"

"What?" she asked.

"I noticed that your daughter breathes through her mouth and not her nose. Chest cold, allergy, or asthma?"

Sandy told me that her daughter, Sarah, had been suffering from asthma since she was a year old. And, at two and a half, she knew where Mommy kept the medicine to help her breathe, which was, of course, an inhalant. Baby Sarah knew how to use it herself, too, since Sandy taught her as a precautionary measure. Sandy said that she had also taught her four-year-old son how to administer the inhalant to Sarah in case of an emergency.

"Unfortunately," continued Sandy, "Sarah is destined to be on this stuff for a long time." Then she added, "Look how tiny she is. All that medication has slowed her growth."

Sarah was smaller than most children her age, and she looked rather pale. I bent down to talk to Sarah, but she backed up to her mother's side and held on to Sandy's skirt. She was obviously very shy.

"Has the doctor considered adding nutrients to her diet, specifically vitamin A?" I asked.

"Bob, are you kidding? I asked him about vitamin C, and he said 'No, not at this time.' Why are doctors so against vitamins? And why are you asking about vitamin A?"

Sarah interrupted us.

"Mommy, my head hurts."

We both looked at little Sarah.

Sandy knelt down on one knee and took Sarah in her arms. "She gets headaches quite often. Poor baby, Mommy will kiss the hurt away." With tears in her eyes, Sandy kissed Sarah on the forehead and then on each side of the head. "There, baby, the pain will go away real soon."

"How often does she have headaches?" I asked.

"It varies. Sometimes not at all, sometimes twice a day, and there are times when she won't have a headache for days. I don't like giving her baby aspirin, but I don't know what else to do. The doctor prescribed two different medicines for Sarah but they make her nauseated. She won't take them because, as she says, 'It puts a bad taste in my mouth.' My poor little girl."

"Is Sarah always so shy or is it just me?"

"She's stressed-out. Between the asthma, sinus problems, wheezing, sneezing, coughing, headaches, nausea, oh my—my little baby has so many things wrong with her. And now she's starting to get nosebleeds."

"What has her doctor said about the nosebleeds?"

"My doctor had me take her to a pediatric specialist who said that it was probably caused by one of the antibiotics, and that I should just put a cold pack on the back of her neck and another on her nose. It works, but I'm not happy with that kind of therapy. Why can't they tell me which antibiotic is causing it and stop prescribing it?"

"Sandy, would you consider including a couple of vitamins in her diet? This would be in addition to, not a replacement for, her regular medication."

"Yes, Bob, I'd consider it because I trust you, but shouldn't I get the doctor's approval first?"

"Of course you should. Anytime anyone is under a doctor's care, he or she should always get the doctor's approval. The final decision is always between you and your doctor."

"What if the doctor says no? After all, he already said not at this time on the vitamin C. Do you think he'll say yes to these two? What two are you talking about?"

"Vitamin A and pantothenic acid. And as for your question about whether or not he'll approve them, my answer is *probably not*—especially the vitamin A, and he most likely will not be familiar with pantothenic acid."

"I'm not either. What is it?"

"Pantothenic acid is vitamin B-5. It's also known as the stress vitamin, or actually the anti-stress vitamin. Some B-5 deficiency symptoms include headaches, sneezing, coughing that is caused by a nasal drip, sinus problems, and, of course, asthma."

"That's everything Sarah has wrong with her."

"No, Sandy, she also has those little bumps on the back of her arms and puffiness under those sweet but sad-looking eyes."

"Bumps? You mean chicken skin? At least that's what the doctor called it."

"The bumps, or chicken skin, are a symptom of a vitamin A deficiency. The puffiness under the eyes could be either a lack of pantothenic acid, vitamin A, or both."

"Bob, how did you know about the bumps on her arms?"

"I suspected that she had them, so I looked. I had to verify my suspicions. Does she have them on the top of her legs as well?"

I got a resounding *yes* from Sandy. "How can I get her to swallow pills? Isn't she too young to swallow? She can chew the baby aspirin, but can she chew these two vitamins?"

"Your daughter can get her vitamin A from cod liver oil, and the B-5 is in a capsule. You can pull apart the capsule and add it to some fruit juice of her choosing. Do you want to consider starting her on them, with doctor's approval, of course?"

Sandy pondered her decision for several moments before deciding. She asked how she could get her daughter to take that awful-tasting cod liver oil.

I told her that today cod liver oil is flavored, and that if she, Sandy, didn't make a face, Sarah would probably like it. When she asked me how long it would take to know if the vitamins were working or would ever work, I knew she had made her decision to try them.

"What about the doctor?" I asked. "What about his approval, or disapproval?"

"It's his disapproval I'm concerned about. I know he will say no, and yet because this could work I have to try. I have to try for Sarah's sake. I know it won't hurt her. Bob, could it interfere with any of her medication?"

"Ask your pharmacist, who will be familiar with contraindications between drugs and vitamins. Sandy, just don't give her these vitamins instead of her medication. They are not a substitute."

Two weeks later Sandy came in after work to tell me that little Sarah enjoyed the cod liver oil, and then asked if it would be okay for her son to take it as well. It seemed as though he had gotten a little jealous of Sarah's taking the orange-flavored drink. Apparently he was able to sneak a taste of Sarah's cod liver oil without his mother's knowing it and liked it. A year later, Sandy would tell me that the pediatrician was surprised that her son hadn't caught any colds the past year and consequently didn't need any antibiotics. But I'm getting ahead of the story... I asked how Sarah was doing.

"Oh, a little better."

"A little better tells me something isn't working. I know that you're giving Sarah the cod liver oil, but what about the B-5? Are you giving her that as well?"

"Well, no, not every day. It's difficult adding a little bit to each glass of orange juice, and so I sometimes skip a day, especially when I'm trying to get the children to the babysitter and myself off to work. I'm not a very good mother, am I?"

"Sandy, you're a terrific and caring mother. Here's an idea that will make giving her the B-5 much easier. Add the entire contents of the capsule to enough orange juice to last for two days. That way, you can give her a small glassful with each meal. Pantothenic acid is a water-soluble vitamin, so taking it throughout the day will enhance its effectiveness."

Sandy reported back the following week. "Bob, I can't believe the difference in Sarah. Her headaches are gone, her sneezing is gone…her…her, oh I can hardly talk I'm so excited! Bob, she's only needed the inhaler two times in the past week! Could it be the vitamins? It must be! She's never gone so long without needing the inhaler. I can't believe it! And no more headaches! I said that already, didn't I?" Sandy gave me a big hug and said, "God bless you."

"Hold it a moment. Yes, it could be the vitamins and thank you for the blessing, but let's wait a little longer before any celebration."

"You're right, Bob, but it has been a very joyous week. I mean, my little baby wheezes only at night and when she gets excited, of course. But she used to wheeze almost throughout the day. What can I expect next? Will she ever be able to throw away her inhaler and all that medicine? Will she ever be cured?"

I first saw little Sarah in August. By Christmas of that year, little Sarah did indeed throw away the inhaler. For the next two years, prior to Sandy and her family moving, Sarah did not need her inhaler. With the doctor's approval, Sandy also discontinued giving Sarah the antibiotics. And, within those next two years Sarah couldn't be called "little" anymore, except affectionately of course, as she grew to be as tall as the others in her preschool class.

42

Nosebleeds

"Hey, you two, how are things in the mountains?" It was a question directed at a mother and her young daughter, who, along with the remainder of the family, had moved there earlier that year.

They assured me that things were great: the weather, the schools, and their new home.

"Did you cut yourself?" I asked the young girl.

"No," answered her mother. "What made you ask that?"

"I noticed she had a crumpled tissue in her hand, and it looked like it had blood on it."

"I get nosebleeds," the young girl said.

"And do you get colds more readily now that you live up in the cold country?"

"No, the rest of us don't, but Janine has had several colds already. She seems to have more problems with her sinuses, too," the mother said.

"Gayle, would you mind rolling up Janine's sleeve? I'd like to look at the back of her arms."

"I don't know if she'll let me. She has these little goose bumps on the backs of them, and the kids at school tease her about them."

"No need for me to see them. How often do you get these nosebleeds?" I directed the question at Janine, who looked at her mother as if to get her okay to answer. Her mother nodded.

"I get them all of the time—even at school. The school nurse said it was a combination of my allergy problems and maybe the start of asthma. So did the doctor."

"And he put you on medication?"

This time the mother answered. "Yes, he put her on an antibiotic for the allergies and a salve that she applies to the inside of her nose. When that didn't work, he cauterized the inside of her nose. That only helped a short while. She still gets the nosebleeds in spite of it all. Bob, do you have an idea?"

"She's probably very deficient in vitamin A. I say that even though too much vitamin A actually causes nosebleeds. In Janine's case, she appears very deficient. I base this on her frequent nosebleeds, her allergies, the many colds, the possibility of respiratory problems, but, in particular, the goose bumps on her arms."

"Why vitamin A? Isn't that the dangerous vitamin?"

"Yes and no. Let me explain the role it plays in the conditions of the nose. The nose is lined with a mucous membrane in which vitamin A plays an integral part. A shortage of this vitamin leads to a dry condition of the mucous membranes."

Gayle interjected, "That's what the doctor said. He didn't mention vitamin A, but he said the lining of her nose was too thin; that's why he prescribed the salve. The antibiotics were for the infection."

"Good, then the doctor and I agree on that. However, in my opinion, vitamin A should be used as the lubricant of the mucous linings rather than the prescribed salve. Vitamin A also provides for the defense of the mucous membranes, which helps in fighting infection."

"You mean, then, that Janine doesn't need the antibiotic?"

"No, that's not what I'm saying. I mean that if she had a sufficient amount of vitamin A in her diet, there might not have been a need for an antibiotic, as there might not have been an infection."

"Let's go with the vitamin A. Does she need any other vitamins?" asked Gayle.

"Gayle, you should also consider the bioflavonoids. They strengthen the microscopic capillaries that are doing the bleeding."

Within the next week, Janine's nosebleeds stopped. As for the asthma, it never did materialize. Her colds lessened to two a year, the goose bumps on her arms disappeared, and her allergies subsided significantly.

43

Plantar Warts

I was waiting on his wife, but I couldn't help notice him. He seemed very uncomfortable, as if in silent pain, and was shifting his weight from one foot to the other. I asked one of my employees to get him a chair while his wife completed her sale.

Then I asked the wife, "Is your husband in pain?"

She looked over at her husband and nodded yes.

Her silence caused me to ask, "He doesn't want to talk about it, does he?"

She nodded again.

A multitude of possible conditions he might be afflicted with were running through my mind. Based on his wife's silent answers, I wondered whether I should pursue the situation any further.

She broke the silence. "He has plantar warts on the soles of his feet."

It was at that moment that my employee Bette delivered the chair to the husband. He thanked her for the chair and then looked over at his wife. Was it with approval or disapproval? I couldn't tell, but was relieved when he smiled at her and asked, "You told him, didn't you?"

"Actually, she didn't. I saw that you seemed uncomfortable, so I asked Bette to bring you a chair. That's when I asked your wife if you were in some kind of pain."

"I need to get these warts burned off again."

"How many do you have and what, besides burning them off, has the doctor prescribed?"

"Initially I had just one, then it multiplied to four, that's when I went to the doctor. He prescribed some kind of salve, which obviously didn't work because the four warts became ten! That's when he decided to cut them off, which did help for awhile, but they always came back, and usually in higher numbers. That's when the doctor decided to try burning them off. Now the warts are on both feet, and the ten warts have become almost countless. It's especially tough for me, because I am a mechanic and stand on my feet all day. If I don't get them burned or cut off, it affects my job performance. Do you have any suggestions?"

"As a matter of fact, I do."

When I told them that "the book" recommended that he take 100,000 units of vitamin A for a month, they both interrupted me by saying, "That much vitamin A is dangerous!"

"It could be, but how much of that high of a potency are you truly assimilating? If you change the dosage each month and also allow for a few days of not taking the vitamin, it will be okay."

I could still see the doubt in their eyes, so I led both of them into the book section of my store and suggested they read about plantar warts in the book *Prescription for Nutritional Healing*. Ten minutes later, they told me to fill their basket with what the doctor had suggested in his book. I did as they asked, and within four months of following the instructions in the book, the husband's warts disappeared. For the next ten plus years that I knew the couple, the husband's plantar warts never returned.

44

Bad Breath

It is difficult to tell people they have bad breath. I'm never sure whether they're already aware of it and, if not, whether my saying so would embarrass them. Is their bad breath caused by something they ate? Is it their teeth or diseased gums? Maybe it's their tonsils or something they drank. I handle this situation as delicately as possible so as not to offend them.

One female customer's breath was atrocious. It didn't appear to be garlic- or onion-related, and I didn't want to get any closer to her than I had to. Was she aware of her bad breath? I asked what I could help her find, and she answered that she wanted a multiple vitamin complex.

"Do you prefer capsules or tablets?"

She answered that all vitamin pills made her sick, so she wasn't sure if our brand was any better than what she had been buying.

"Sick in what way?" I needed to get answers from her to determine the cause of her bad breath. Maybe she'd just eaten. She may have had garlic, onions, or another odorous herb in her food, although her breath did not smell like garlic. Her breath smelled like something dead.

"Oh, I get nauseated. It's like I have to burp a lot more."

"What do you mean, a lot more? Do you have more than the usual upper gas after eating?"

I received a resounding yes! Not only did she burp a lot, but she could taste it as well.

"Have you been checked for this problem? I mean, have you been to your doctor for a diagnosis?"

"Oh yeah, I saw him. He told me to take an over-the-counter antacid and breath mints, but they only helped a little, and then they didn't work at all. I still take them, though, because I don't know what else to do."

I asked if she had been to her dentist or if she had sinus problems, but neither the dentist nor the doctor diagnosed her as having any problem in those areas. I then asked her several questions regarding hydrochloric acid. I got affirmatives on all of the questions I asked, which meant she was probably lacking this important digestive aid. One of the questions regarding a hydrochloric acid deficiency is: "Do you have bad breath?" Her *yes* to the question enabled me to talk more freely about her breath. After explaining the actions and benefits of hydrochloric acid and a product called acidophilus, she decided to buy them both.

As she was leaving the store, she asked, "Acidophilus before I eat and the other when I eat. Why can't I just take them at the same time?"

"Do you want relief or not?"

45

Bad Breath and the Sinuses

Bad breath has many causes, so recommending any one remedy before some investigation is not advisable.

Max, a middle-aged man who was always laughing, had very bad breath, a problem that was compounded by the smell traveling in every direction. He had been to the medical doctors, but when they checked his stomach they could not find a cause for this bad breath, or halitosis. Max had been to several other vitamin stores and even a nutritional doctor, all to no avail. When he came into our store for the first time, I greeted him with my usual "Happy Thursday" (or whatever day it happened to be).

This inspired him to laugh as he said hello, and I got the full brunt of his really bad breath. It was truly disgusting. Fortunately, I didn't have to address his breath problem, as he was the one who brought it up.

He asked, "Can you help me with my halitosis?"

I asked the usual questions: "Have you been to a doctor? What was the diagnosis? Are you on medication? Have you been to a dentist?"

Max said he had seen them all but that no one was able to determine the cause of his problem. He had tried breath mints, chlorophyll, acidophilus, parsley, enzymes, hydrochloric acid (a naturally occurring stomach acid in pill form), and even chewing gum. They all helped for a short while, but not one of them corrected the problem. I had to look deeper to find a solution. I noticed that he tilted his head from side to side as he spoke; this prompted questions related to a deficiency of pantothenic acid. His several *yeses* to my questions caused me to query him about vitamin A, and he appeared deficient in this, too. Yes to both. Now I asked, "How bad is your sinus problem?"

"Oh, it always bothers me. Can you fix that too?"

"I don't deal with specific health problems; I deal with correcting nutritional deficiencies. If correcting a deficiency corrects your diagnosed problem, good. That means there was a correlation and we got lucky."

It appeared that his halitosis was caused by the problem with his sinuses. By correcting his deficiencies of pantothenic acid and vitamin A, perhaps his halitosis would be corrected as well.

"That's a strange and different approach. Wouldn't it be great if you fixed both my sinus problem and my bad breath problem? My wife would love you for it. In fact, she won't sleep with me anymore because of both my labored breathing and my bad breath."

Max continued with the acidophilus and enzymes and added vitamin A, pantothenic acid, and colloidal silver nasal spray from Sovereign Silver to his vitamin regimen. His sinuses were the first to clear up, and within one week, his breath became more bearable. I saw him a couple of months later. He was laughing just as much, or perhaps, even more, because his laughter no longer included a wave of bad breath. Now he considered his breath and breathing normal. His wife agreed wholeheartedly. So did I.

46

Gas - Upper and Lower

One afternoon I was an invited guest at someone else's family get-together. The homemade food was wonderful. It was a fun-filled afternoon until Tony, Big Uncle Tony, began his interpretation of the tuba. Everyone ran. No, Uncle Tony doesn't play a musical instrument. He has terrible gas, and he doesn't care where he releases it. In my opinion, both Tony and the odor were obnoxious. Unfortunately, the family had accepted Uncle Tony and, as they called it, his playing of the tuba. I was asked by one of the family members if there was something that could be done about Uncle Tony.

"Yes, have him go see a medical doctor and find out what's wrong with him, besides his manners."

Tony responded in retaliation to my remark with, "There's nothing wrong with me except that everything I eat turns to gas. The family has accepted my condition."

I didn't apologize for what I had said about his manners because I believed his actions, although funny to him and accepted by the family, were crude and selfish. I was asked again, this time by Tony's wife, if I could do or suggest something that would help her husband. Since Tony wasn't interested, I decided to talk to his wife and ask her about Tony's problem.

Whenever there is a condition that appears to be related to a stomach problem, I always ask if a medical doctor has checked that person, in case it has anything to do with the heart. No, Tony's ailment was not associated with his heart. I then ask questions related to hydrochloric acid.

"Yes, yes, yes! That's my Tony," she answered, and her two children echoed their mom's response. "Yes, that's Dad…So, can something be done?" they asked in unison.

I answered, "Yes, and if Tony is agreeable, I could offer relief for his symptoms."

Reluctantly Tony said yes, which was mostly due to the chorus of relatives egging him on. He took three hydrochloric acid pills from the bottle and swallowed them down without drinking any liquid. Uncle Tony was all show.

"That's my Uncle Tony. He doesn't need any liquid."

"Unless it's a beer," chimed in another. Everyone laughed.

"Now what?" asked Tony. "What happens next? How will I know if this stuff is working?"

I responded, "As far as the upper gas is concerned, you'll know right away, certainly within the hour. The lower gas will take a few hours or a couple of days. That depends on the transit time of your food, meaning the time it takes from eating a meal to the elimination of that same meal through a bowel movement."

Of course, Tony was annoyed with the latter answer. After a couple of hours, Uncle Tony did indeed stop burping. Even he was amazed. The hydrochloric acid had stopped the buildup of gas in his stomach, which helped with his upper intestinal gas problem.

"Is he cured?" I was asked.

"No, this is just the beginning," I answered, knowing Tony needed more than the three hydrochloric acid pills he had just taken. I handed Tony's wife some more pills for Tony to take with dinner and dessert later on that day. I then said my goodbyes to the family and was glad to be away from Tony.

Two days later, Tony's wife called me at my store. "Tony hasn't had any real gas since late last night after taking the rest of the pills you gave me. Is he all better? What does he do next?"

I suggested that Tony come into one of our stores, take the Body Language Questionnaire, and return it to me for an evaluation.

"You mean he might have to take these pills forever?"

"Probably. Unless he starts making some changes in his eating and drinking habits," I cautioned.

"I'll tell Tony what you said."

We said our goodbyes.

Later that day, Tony's wife called again. "Tony said he's not about to take any more pills. The family is going to have to accept him as he is, and if they don't they're not family."

I wish every story had a happy ending. This one, because of Tony's attitude, didn't end well. Although I never saw Tony or his family again, I heard that he's just as obnoxious as ever, except now he has developed ulcers and a hiatal hernia. It was inevitable, due to his lack of hydrochloric acid.

47

Looking at Teeth

I was washing some fingerprints off the outside of the door when a woman drove up and parked her car in front of my store. As she got out of the car she commented, "Oh, and you do windows too."

I grinned and added, "Yes, but only once a year and this happened to be that day."

I held the door open for her to enter.

She thanked me and said, "This is my first time in this store. I usually shop at, well, somewhere else but my hairdresser told me about your store and so here I am."

At this point I usually ask what one is looking for, but this time I said, "Excuse me for asking what might be an embarrassing question, but do you have any digestive problems? I mean, do you have bloating or a full feeling after eating? Perhaps more than the usual upper gas such as burping or belching?" I hoped I hadn't overwhelmed or offended her with these questions. After all, this was her first time at our store and she didn't really know how we did business.

"Why did you ask me about digestive problems? What gave you any indication that I might, and I emphasize *might,* have a digestion problem?"

I quickly offered her an apology, but instead of accepting it she just continued asking the same question. "Why did you ask me about a possible digestive problem?" she repeated.

I explained to her how our bodies sort of "talk" about possible deficiencies we might have. Most people do not know how to interpret these body signals and usually ignore or accept them as part of growing older. Most doctors aren't aware of these bodily signs either.

"Okay, okay, I accept your reason and I accept your apology, but why, I mean what so-called body sign did I give you to ask me about digestion?"

"Your teeth. Actually, your lack of teeth. When you were talking I noticed that your back molars are missing. Both upper and lower. This could mean that you're not chewing your food as thoroughly as you should, and that could result in digestive problems. So there, I'm caught and I plead guilty."

"Are you Bob?" she asked.

I answered yes.

"Bob, I've been going both to a medical doctor and a chiropractor, and for the past four months have not been able to figure out why I have, as you guessed, digestive problems. And you, in less than five minutes, no, less than two minutes, not only determined that I have a problem but you also discovered the cause. Or at the least, the possible cause. My hairdresser was right, you are amazing."

"Thank you for saying all of those nice things, but it was just a guess. Now we have to find out if your missing teeth point to the cause."

I offered her the Body Language Questionnaire and through her answers determined that she was indeed deficient in enzymes and hydrochloric acid. Both of these are instrumental in helping digestion and assimilation of food. She wanted to buy them both.

"Whoa, not so fast. As important as these items are, they're not going to cure your problem. That's going to require some dental work."

"I guess I put off going to the dentist for too long. I promise myself and you that I will set up an appointment when I get home today. I promise. I just don't like the hurting associated with dentistry. Thank you for your help and thanks for these two items."

She picked up the bag containing the enzymes and hydrochloric acid and started for the door.

"There's more," I said.

"What else do I have to buy?"

"Nothing. You're going to have to adopt a new approach to eating."

She set her bag down and asked, smiling, "Do I need to take notes?"

I returned the smile and told her how she needed to pre-cut her food, especially the meat products, into small pieces—very small pieces. This would enable her to chew these pieces more thoroughly even though she would be only using her remaining front teeth. Next, stop drinking liquids with, or immediately after eating. Drink just enough to swallow down the pills she had just bought.

"But I feel that I need liquid to get the food down," was her retort.

"Did you know that one produces a liter of saliva each day? Almost a quart. That should be enough liquid to get your food down. How to generate this liquid is by chewing, even with the limited teeth you have. If you chew long enough, adequate saliva will be produced. Saliva, besides being an enzyme itself, also acts as a lubricant for food to pass through the throat and into the stomach."

Although she was not taking notes, I could see she was accepting my suggestions.

It took only two days for her to correct her digestive problems. Eventually, she did get partial dentures to replace her missing back teeth, and she continued her newly established eating habits. She didn't suffer from another digestive problem for the next two years that she remained a customer.

48

You Can't Help Me!

I had only been in business a few months when an older guy (I was much younger then) came into my store just at closing time. I greeted him and asked how I could help him.

"Help me?" he asked. "You can't help me. The only thing you can do is sell me some vitamin E. I have experts helping me."

Experts? I thought. *Should I pursue his statement or forget about it?* He seemed cantankerous, it was already closing time, and I didn't particularly want to get into a discussion about something he had already made up his mind about. "Forget it, Bob," I said to myself. Then it happened, my curiosity caused me to ask, "What kind of experts?" There, I did it. I opened up a conversation I knew would waste our time, and I wanted to get home for dinner.

He looked at me and said, "Experts, not clerks. Experts, as in the best of the best doctors. I'm seeing my personal doctor, who is an internist. At his suggestion, I'm also seeing a cardiologist, a gastrointestinal doctor, and a surgeon, who also specializes in the removal of hemorrhoids. They're my experts. I don't need anymore. From you, I just need the vitamin E."

"A very impressive array of experts," I lied. I handed him a bottle of vitamin E and then asked, "Let's see, the cardiologist because of your heart—that would be obvious. The GI specialist because of ulcers, I presume. Or is it irritable bowel syndrome?"

He nodded yes and was about to say something, but I continued talking before he could interject.

"And the surgeon, of course, to operate on your hemorrhoids. What about your ulcers, will he operate on them as well?" I waited for his answer, but now he seemed to be ignoring my questions. He turned the vitamin E bottle around as he read the label. Still ignoring my questions, he opened up the conversation by asking me about vitamin E. He asked me the difference between the natural versus the synthetic, the difference between alpha tocopherol and mixed tocopherol, and a capsule versus a tablet. As he was talking I noticed his teeth, or rather his lack of teeth. He had, perhaps, six upper teeth and six lower teeth. All incisors, no molars, nothing with which to chew his food. I couldn't help myself.

"These experts, I mean these doctors that you are going to, are they giving you results, good results? After all, as you said, they are the best of the best." I said it without being sarcastic.

"I'm getting results and now they want to cut on me. They said that's what I need to do, get some operations. I trust them."

"Because they're the best," I answered. This time I was just a little sarcastic.

"They are the best!" he retorted.

"How long have you been seeing them?" I was going in for the kill.

"Oh, several months now."

"In my opinion, as a vitamin clerk, of course, you are seeing the wrong doctors, all of them." I looked right at him, waiting for his response.

His eyes narrowed, he took a deep breath and swallowed.

Here it comes, I thought.

"What do you mean, I'm seeing the wrong doctors? They're the best!" he said somewhat angrily.

"You should be seeing a doctor of dentistry. Most likely he, more than the others, would be able to fix your problem without the operations and without most of the medication you, I presume, are taking. These 'best of the very best' should have mentioned the correlation between dentistry and health."

We talked. No, I talked and he listened, and rather intently to what I had to say for a full half-hour. I told him that, in my opinion, not chewing food thoroughly can lead to digestive problems. Having digestive problems means that the medications usually prescribed make the stomach alkaline; in other words, they remove the acid, specifically hydrochloric acid. Without adequate stomach acid, bacteria grow in the stomach and can cause ulcers. A lack of acid does not allow for protein to be absorbed, and protein is needed for the rebuilding of the body, every part of the body, including the entire alimentary canal. If protein is not properly broken down in the stomach, it can lead to putrefaction in the colon, which affects the entire body in one way or another.

"Do you have bad breath?" I asked.

"You seem to have all of the answers, including this one. Yes, I do."

Many times what is diagnosed as a heart condition is a digestive problem.

He interrupted my train of thought. "That's why they don't exactly know what's wrong with my heart. I get lots of pain in my left shoulder. The cardiologist said it's my heart. He's giving me different kinds of medication, but none of them has worked. Do you think it could really be my stomach instead of my heart?"

"Ask your GI doctor, that's his specialty."

The ringing of the telephone interrupted our discussion. It was my wife wanting to know when I would be home, as dinner was ready to be served. As I said goodbye to her, he looked up at our clock and said that he hadn't realized how late it was.

He apologized for keeping me so long past closing time, reached into his wallet, and took out some money to pay for the vitamin E. I offered him the Body Language Questionnaire. He took it, glanced at each page and then folded it and put it in his bag along with his purchase.

"Thank you, really. I mean, thank you very much. I will be back, but first I'm going to find a dentist. I'm tired of having my mouth hurt. I guess I need dentures, but I was afraid to face reality. You've convinced me that my health is more important than my ego. Thank you again."

Over the next several months his health improved as dramatically as his attitude. All I did was make him aware of another avenue to reach better health. It was through his own efforts that he gained back his health.

49

HIATAL HERNIA

"What flavor of ice cream did you have so early in the morning?" I asked my customer after showing him the multiple vitamin section of my store.

"Ice cream? I haven't had any ice cream this morning. Why do you ask?" he countered.

"I noticed, as we were talking, that your tongue was somewhat coated. I was joking about the ice cream, but dairy products do leave a residue on the tongue. Even adding milk to morning coffee can have the same coating effect."

"Yes, I had my morning coffee, but I drink it black. I haven't had any dairy products this morning. My tongue is always coated. My dentist said to brush my tongue whenever I brush my teeth."

"Doesn't help it, does it?"

"Hmmm, I guess only for a short while and then the coating comes back."

"Do you have stomach ulcers or just indigestion?"

"No. I don't have ulcers, although the doctor said I am a candidate for getting them. I guess I worry too much."

"Or drink too many liquids with your meals."

"Too many liquids? Aren't we supposed to drink eight glasses of liquid a day?"

"That's an ideal amount of liquid, but that total doesn't include coffee, just water. I asked you about indigestion. Do you have difficulty digesting food?"

"You keep pushing me for an answer regarding my digestion. What makes you think I have a digestive problem?"

"I'm getting nosey again. I apologize. To answer your question, I'll point out what I noticed when I looked at you. First, I noticed that your tongue was coated. This could have been caused by the consumption of dairy products; however, you said that you hadn't had any milk or ice cream this morning. Next, your age—I would guess that you are at least thirty-five."

"You're kind. I'm fifty-five, and, yes, I do have digestive problems. In fact, the doctors call it a hiatal hernia. I've had it for about six years, with only brief episodes of it getting any better."

"Is your reflux, or regurgitation of food back into the esophagus, caused by a gas buildup in the stomach?"

"Yes. First I eat, and about half an hour or so later I start to have a gas buildup in my stomach. Then I bloat, and soon thereafter I have reflux, then the discomfort, and eventually the accompanying pain. It sounds like you're familiar with this affliction."

"Yes, I am. I used to be in the pharmaceutical industry, and at that time I introduced one of the most popular anti-hiatal-hernia products on the market.

It was designed to act as a barrier so that the gas could not push stomach acid through the cardiac sphincter and into the esophagus. The medical profession accepted it as a boon to their profession."

"What was the name of the product?" he asked.

After I told him the name, he said that he had taken it at one time and thought it was reasonably effective.

"Yes, it did work, and when I got into the vitamin industry, I was concerned that no nutritional product existed that was just as effective. Was I wrong! When I asked some nutritionally oriented doctors what would work to relieve the effects of a hiatal hernia, they explained it to me this way.

"After a person reaches about thirty-two years of age, the digestive system becomes less reliable and starts faltering. This is usually caused by the fact that most people eat too fast and drink too many liquids with their meals. Eating and drinking patterns, combined with daily stress, cause the amount of usable hydrochloric acid in the stomach to decrease. This acid, which naturally occurs in the stomach, is necessary to break proteins down into amino acids and enables the assimilation of certain minerals, especially iron and calcium. Gas forms when sugar and bacteria are combined in the warmth of the stomach. This sugar is not only table sugar, but also the sugar from the foods classified as carbohydrates, including pasta, bread, and, of course, donuts. This gas causes the stomach to bloat, thus pushing the partially ingested food into the esophagus. The medical profession attempts to determine what to do with the gas that has built up in the stomach. In our industry, our goal is to keep the gas from forming in the first place. It's that simple."

He interrupted me by asking, "I forgot to tell you, I also get heartburn, lots of it. According to the doctor, heartburn is caused by too much acid."

"Question: If you were working on your automobile and inadvertently spilled some battery acid on your hand, what would you do first?" I asked.

"Cry out with pain! I've done it, and it really burns."

"After you cried out, what did you do next?"

"I ran for the garden hose and applied water."

"Did that help?"

"Of course."

"Why?"

"Because I diluted the battery acid with water. That stopped the burning."

"Did you ever try that with heartburn? I mean, when you have heartburn, which as you said was "too much acid," did you try drinking a glass of water to dilute the acid?"

"Yes, but it didn't work."

"Why do you suppose?"

"I don't know. Maybe it's a different kind of acid—one that can't be diluted with water."

"According to the nutritional doctors, the heartburn may have originated because you didn't have enough hydrochloric acid, rather than too much. Let me continue with their story.

"These nutritional doctors said that to stop the effects of a hiatal hernia, we must keep the gas from forming. Their reasoning is that another main function of hydrochloric acid is to destroy bacteria in the stomach so they don't enter into the small intestines. If hydrochloric acid destroys the bacteria in the stomach, and bacteria is one of the three ingredients that create gas, the buildup of gas is prevented. Thus, no gas buildup and no reflux. It has also been determined that ulcers are caused by bacteria. If there was an adequate amount of hydrochloric acid to begin with, it would have destroyed the bacteria before the bacteria caused the ulcer."

"This sounds like I need more acid in my stomach, rather than that I have too much. I'm being treating for too much acid, which makes no sense if I actually need more acid for good digestion."

"It will cost you about seven dollars to determine whose theory is correct."

"How's that?"

"Buy some hydrochloric acid and try it."

"When and how will I know if it works?"

"If you take it according to the instructions on the bottle with tonight's dinner and reduce your fluid intake with your meal, you should know within an hour or two after eating."

"What if I get heartburn from the increased acid?"

"What did you do when you got the battery acid on your hand?"

"Sounds too simple, but I'll try it."

He called the next day and asked if hydrochloric acid was available in a larger bottle.

50

ECZEMA

A connection exists between fats and oils and health and disease. Some people, although overweight, are actually deficient in fat—friendly fat, that is. * They could lack friendly fats in their diet or, due to a digestive problem, be unable to assimilate these fats. Such was the case of Augie. Unfortunately, he suffered from an obvious deficiency of friendly fat and, as I was soon to learn, was not able to absorb the small amount of friendly fat he was getting in his diet.

I first saw Augie as the husband of a customer. He was standing outside my store reading a newspaper while his wife was inside shopping. I couldn't help wondering if he was actually reading the paper or hiding his face in it. I had caught a quick glimpse of his face. My guess was that, because of the severity of his condition, he was too embarrassed to enter my store, so he waited outside. I had to find out about his malady, so I walked outside to greet him.

"Good morning."

He didn't answer.

"Any good news today?" I asked.

He still didn't answer.

It was obvious he didn't want to talk to me, and I certainly didn't want to alienate him and lose his wife as a customer. *Should I risk asking him another question?* I thought. Once again my nosiness got the better of me, so I decided to approach him once more. This time I walked within inches of him.

"Excuse me."

He lowered the newspaper and peered over the top. I couldn't tell whether he was angry with me, because his eyes were hidden behind dark sunglasses. I always look at people's eyes because they are great indicators of emotion, and I could only guess that at this moment, because I was obviously annoying him, his eyes would reveal some anger. Anger at me. But I also suspected that beyond this look of anger, his eyes would reveal pain and suffering because of his condition.

"You're not going to acknowledge me, are you?"

He raised the newspaper, covering his face again. In a raspy voice he answered, "My wife does the shopping, not me."

"Your wife is being taken care of. It's you whom I need to ask some questions. What is the problem with your face?" Was the question too impertinent, too bold?

"I have no problem with my face. It's you that I have a problem with." He lowered the newspaper, revealing his entire face.

His statement was a challenge I couldn't back away from.

"Look, I know I'm being a pest, and I'm not here to start a fight. I want to see if I can help you."

"Nobody can help me. Even the best of the best doctors."

"When you say 'doctors,' does that mean you're seeing dermatologists?"

He nodded and then took off his glasses. I was hoping that didn't mean he was going to throw a punch at me.

"They've tried creams, ointments, lotions, and, most recently, peeling off my skin. Does it look as if their therapy is working? And they're supposed to be the best in Los Angeles. Now you want to see if you can help me. Back off, young man, I've given up."

He put his sunglasses on, brought the newspaper up to cover his face, and turned away from me. I was obviously dismissed.

This was one of the worst cases of dermatitis I had ever seen. His face looked like a chunk of raw meat that had been pounded by a meat cleaver. There were holes, pockmarks, and a pus-like liquid oozing from his forehead and the sides of his face. The disease had spread into his ears and eyelids and was circling his mouth. I stood there for a moment longer and then re-entered the store. I refused to give up on him, but would I be able to convince him that there might be some help here? Not a cure, of course—I wasn't so arrogant to think that nutrients could save the world. But if there was just the slightest relief, just a lessening of the pain, I had to follow through, and I had to keep the potential remedy simple and effective. I picked up a bottle of liquid lecithin, put it in a bag, and walked outside to where he was standing.

"Hi. It's me again, the pest."

He turned slowly and lowered the newspaper.

"Look, I have no idea as to the pain and suffering you are going through, but do me a favor, even though you don't owe me one. I need to know if this stuff works on a case as severe as yours. If it does, it will be a big help to others I know who are hurting from a similar problem. If this liquid remedy doesn't work...well, I'll be very sorry. But give it a chance. Give me a chance too. Prove me right or prove me wrong."

"Nonsense. Vitamins are nonsense."

"Do you realize that you just decreased the effectiveness of this product?"

"I did what?"

"Decreased the effectiveness of this product, this gift of Nature. If you don't believe it will work, it lessens the chance of its working by almost 30 percent. Unfortunately, that increases your chance of proving that I am wrong. Now I'm really at a disadvantage, but I'm still willing to challenge you as to its effectiveness. Take it. It's free. The only cost to you is some time and effort." I handed him the bottle and was surprised that he took it from me. I was doubly surprised when he started to read the label.

"Take one tablespoon with each meal and again at bedtime," I said over my shoulder as I turned to go back into the store. Then I heard him call out to me.

"What does it taste like?"

"The taste doesn't matter; it's what it will do for you that's important." My answer sounded too abrupt, so I turned and said, with a smile, that it tasted like walnuts. Then, passing his wife in the doorway, I went into the store. She looked perplexed.

Wait, wait, wait. That's always the toughest part of a situation like this. Would he even consider doing as I suggested? It was three days before he telephoned me.

"This lecithin stuff, does it give you diarrhea?"

The only thing that raced through my mind was that he was taking the lecithin. And that meant he had not given up and was trying my suggestion.

The delay in my answering caused him to ask the question again. I answered with another question. "Do you usually have constipation?"

"Yeah, something terrible. The odor is awful, too."

I simply cannot describe what I was feeling inside. It was a mixture of excitement, satisfaction, relief, and joy. But mostly I was getting answers about the possible cause, or causes, of his dermatitis. Perhaps he would eventually give me the time to counsel him nutritionally through the Body Language Questionnaire.

"Yes, lecithin could cause diarrhea, especially with the amount you're taking. But continue with the four tablespoons a day because loose bowels do contribute to the cleansing of one's system."

Constant diarrhea is not good for the body, as it leads to mineral deficiencies and an electrolyte imbalance. Since I had given him a quart bottle of lecithin, I knew that this condition couldn't last for more than a week. As for his skin problem, I didn't need to know if there was any improvement, my satisfaction was in knowing that he cared enough to try. We hung up without discussing it.

The following Saturday one of my employees called for me to come up front, saying there was someone there to see me. What I saw, I hadn't expected. I even asked myself if this was the same man I had given the lecithin to a week earlier. He walked toward me, extending his hand. His face, although still very inflamed, had a smile from ear to ear. As he took my hand into his, the tears began streaming down his face. He pulled me closer and wrapped his other arm around me into a bear hug.

We do a lot of hugging at my store, but this hug was special. Here was a man who had almost given up on his life and within a week had made the effort to change it. After he let me loose, he proudly showed me the improvement in his condition. Now, he *wanted* to show me his face!

"Look, look at my eyelids. They're almost completely well. I can open and close my eyes without pain. And my ears—they're clearing up, too. I can't believe it. I just can't believe it. No, I'm not going to show you up my nose, but now I can blow it without pain."

He was laughing and crying. "My face, I used to call it one big, oozing blister. I couldn't laugh, I couldn't smile, and now I can do both."

He carefully wiped his cheeks. "And now I can painlessly cry with joy instead of with distress."

I looked around at those watching us and noticed that there wasn't a dry eye amongst them all, including me. It was a very touching moment.

After the situation settled down, I gave him a Body Language Questionnaire and asked that he complete it at home and bring it back for my computer evaluation. I would do a more in-depth nutritional counseling based on the results.

The outcome of his questionnaire helped me determine that Augie (we finally introduced ourselves) was deficient in many nutrients. Additionally, he couldn't tolerate spicy foods, was overweight, had constipation, didn't sleep well, and his body seemed to be unable to assimilate oils, which are necessary for the lubrication of the body.

Augie did a gallbladder cleanse, enabling him to assimilate oils readily and lessening his sensitivity to spicy food. His deficiency of the mineral magnesium contributed to the constipation problem and the irregular sleep pattern. After taking this supplement for just a few days, both of those issues were remedied. A regular bowel movement was also beneficial in the cleansing of his intestinal tract, which diminished the resorption of toxins into the bloodstream. Before the cleanse, these toxins would have been excreted through his skin, exacerbating his present condition. Although Augie never did attain a 100 percent cure, he did enjoy radical improvement.

At the time this story took place, the only nutrients available to me to remedy conditions such as Augie's included lecithin, safflower oil, vitamins A, C, and E, and cod liver oil. Successes did take place in those early days, but today, with the advent of an almost endless list of oils and other nutrients, the improvement rate has increased dramatically.

My approach to clients, for the most part, is not to be nosey or obnoxious—well, maybe a little nosey! In Augie's situation, I had to be both. But when I asked him how he felt about my behavior he said, "Thanks to you and your industry, I'll never have to hide behind a newspaper and dark glasses again."

*To distinguish the differences between friendly fat and unfriendly fat, I suggest reading *Fats and Oils* by Udo Erasmus.

51

ARTHRITIS

During my second year in the nutrition industry, we didn't have available the glucosamines, MSM, amino acids, or even vitamin C in a potency higher than 500 mg. In those days, we did the best we could with what we had. Despite our limited resources, there were many success stories. This story is one of the most touching to me.

"Good afternoon, young lady. How may I help you?" I inquired.

"Honey, I'm eighty-three. Don't call me 'young lady' unless you're at least a hundred years old. And you're certainly not," she retorted with a smile. "I'm looking for that awful-tasting psyllium stuff. Can't stand the taste but it keeps me regular."

"Capsules or powder?"

"Pills don't work. Need the powder," she said matter-of-factly.

"Have you considered cod liver oil?"

"What for?"

"For your crippling arthritis," I could have said but didn't. This woman's fingers, her curved spine, and the limited ability to walk revealed the severity of the arthritis that ravaged her diminutive body. Her fingers were pointed in every direction except straight. Her knuckles were so badly swollen that she wore her rings as a fine-jeweled necklace. I couldn't even imagine the pain and suffering she must have had. Her body was deformed by arthritis, and I couldn't wait to somehow tell her the story of Doreen.

"If you're not in too much of a hurry, I would like to tell you the story of one of my customers, Doreen. I met Doreen about a year ago as she was completing her purchase right where you're standing. As she was writing the check, I looked at her handwriting, which flowed from one letter to the next like a butterfly kissing each flower it touched. It was so beautiful I couldn't help complimenting her. She stopped writing, looked up at me, and with a very broad and friendly smile thanked me, and then told me she had only been writing for a year and a half, due to crippling arthritis."

At this my customer exclaimed, "Crippling arthritis? It couldn't have been all that bad if she was able to write."

"That's what I thought, too. In fact, I was astonished at her statement. Doreen stood straight, walked straight, and her fingers were straight. She had no visible signs of any arthritis, particularly crippling, and I told her so, but she only smiled and continued telling her story.

"Doreen told me that for many years she had even been confined to a wheelchair. She couldn't walk, stand, or even feed herself because her arms were locked at the elbows. People had to dress her, undress her, and bathe her. She said she had been totally helpless. Day after day, all she could do was watch television. The pain was continuous. It never stopped except for the hour or two when, and if, the pain pill worked. She had lost her desire to live, but even if she had wanted to die she was unable to take her own life because of the paralysis."

My customer interrupted the story.

"She shouldn't even think about taking her life. Life is a gift from God and taking it is not an option. Go ahead, son, I didn't mean to interrupt you."

I smiled and went on with Doreen's story. "One day as she was watching television, she saw a program with Dr. Dale Alexander as the guest. He inspired her so much that she gained hope, the will to live again, which eventually gave her back her life.

"Dr. Alexander was the great promoter of cod liver oil, and he told of its healing powers, especially in arthritis, even crippling arthritis. She cried as she watched the program, inwardly hoping and praying that what he said could help even her. She couldn't wait to tell her children when they got home from work. Her son-in-law was the skeptic, but her two daughters were delighted because they saw, for the first time in many years, a look of hope in her face, in her eyes, and heard it in her voice.

"Her family agreed to go along with her request. She didn't know if they supported this idea because of her attitude change, or perhaps it was just to patronize her, or maybe it was out of sheer desperation. That night she had her first cod liver oil cocktail. She didn't mind the taste too much. If it worked, the taste wouldn't matter."

"What does it taste like? I don't like fish. Does it taste like fish?"

"Cod liver oil is derived from fish, the liver of cod fish, but you can mix it with orange juice or milk. As Doreen said, 'If it works, the taste won't matter.'

After she took her first cocktail, the pain didn't stop, but she felt inside that she was getting better. The next morning, she had her second cocktail and, according to Dr. Alexander's instruction, had another just before bedtime. Dr. Alexander recommends that the morning cocktail be taken first thing in the morning on an empty stomach. Initially, Doreen chose to mix the oil with milk, but over the years she varied it with orange juice. After drinking the cocktail, she had to wait, again according to Dr. Alexander, at least a half-hour before the next cocktail, which was water. But it had to be reasonably hot water and, once again, the hot water was to be taken on an empty stomach. Then she waited one hour before eating breakfast."

"Honey, that sure seems like an awful lot of bother. Anyway, I like eating my toast and having my coffee just after waking up," said my new customer.

"Doreen used to eat toast and coffee, but switched to old-fashioned oatmeal. Sometimes she added raisins for variety. In Dr. Alexander's opinion, sugar was white poison so she stopped using it and switched to honey. According to Dr. Alexander, honey is a good substitute but it, too, should be used in moderation. Dr. Alexander recommended that the nighttime cocktail be consumed three hours after the evening meal, using the same procedure as with the morning cocktail. Again, this involved first the cod liver oil and, a half-hour later, the hot water. Probably the first positive reaction Doreen experienced was being able to sleep longer than the usual two hours, at which time she would need another pain pill. Over the next few weeks, her need for pain pills diminished to less than half."

"I don't know how she could do that. My doctor said I would be on pain pills forever," my customer interjected.

"Doreen's doctor, too, was a skeptic, and warned her to continue with the pain pills so as not to put her body into shock. Her doctor truly believed that she was faking about experiencing less pain and that her improvement was all psychological. He believed the pain was still there, but that she just wouldn't admit to it. He finally changed his mind, however, when she showed him 50 percent improvement in the movements of her fingers and arms. The doctor was finally convinced and decided to restart her therapy.

"Doreen's daughters were elated when she showed them she was able to stand, although she still had to hold on to something or someone. All these improvements took place after only eight months of taking the cod liver oil cocktails. At first she only *believed* she would be able to walk again, but after her many successes her attitude changed. Now she *knew* she would walk. After her daughter bought Dr. Alexander's arthritis cookbook, there were many changes made in her diet. His cookbook had numerous recipes that Doreen had her daytime nurse's aide prepare. Her nurse, who at first was a non-believer, eventually changed her own attitude and started doing the morning cocktail along with Doreen. She even ate Dr. Alexander's menus. It appeared that everybody's life was changing and for the better. One of the most touching statements Doreen made to me was that, except for her Bible, his book became the book she most read. When her daughter offered to buy a new edition, Doreen told her no, she had highlighted everything that was important to her, and if she had a new book, she'd have to do the highlighting all over again."

My customer was smiling, but I wasn't so sure she was listening to what I was saying. I wanted to convince her to try the cod liver oil, so I went on with the story.

"Within two years of starting the program, Doreen was walking, albeit with two canes, but she emphasized that she was walking. After two more years, she "retired the canes." Her wheelchair had been given to a local nursing home, but her daughter wanted to keep the canes—just in case. The canes, too, were eventually donated to the same nursing home. After five years on the cod liver oil cocktails, Doreen regained over 90 percent use of her fingers, hands, arms, legs, and neck. And now her whole body was working again. She recalled how thrilled she was when she was able to turn the first page in Dr. Alexander's book all by herself. She cried because, before, turning a page had been an impossible task. Imagine crying over something as simple as that. No time for crying anymore because now, as she says it so nicely, "I am happy with my life and realize how precious it is."

"Cod liver oil comes in two flavors, orange and mint. Which flavor do you want?" I asked my customer.

"Honey, that was a very sweet story, but for me to take cod liver oil, no way. I don't care what the flavor is, it still would taste like fish oil, and I can't stand the taste of fish oil." She hobbled out of the store.

"Twelve seconds," I said loudly, although she didn't hear me. "Twelve seconds twice a day versus twenty-four hours of continuous pain." I felt such a great sadness for this woman. I could only hope and pray that maybe someday she would change her mind and consider the cod liver oil cocktail.

A few weeks later, I saw Doreen across the street from my store. She was running from her car and into a shoe store. I said aloud, "Look at that lady run."

The three customers who were in my store at the time looked at Doreen and then back at me. They were probably thinking, "Why wouldn't she run—after all, it is raining outside."

Because of the rain, these customers were a captive audience, so I told them the Doreen story, too.

Betsy, one of the customers, bought some cod liver oil for her own arthritic condition. Although her problem wasn't as severe as Doreen's or the other customer in this story, she could barely hold a knife or fork without spilling food. She, too, was receiving medication for pain. She followed the same regimen as Doreen, including making dietary changes. After several weeks of cod liver oil cocktails, the severity of Betsy's joint pain decreased enough that she was able to sleep through most of the night. Her fingers were becoming more flexible, and her wrists were less inflamed.

Early one Monday afternoon, Betsy and her husband visited me at the store. They were both eating ice cream cones. For her husband that was okay, but for Betsy it was totally contrary to what I had been preaching about high-sugar foods. I guess I get more involved with my customers than I realize; I told them I was disheartened to see them eating ice cream.

That's when Betsy's husband interrupted me mid-sentence saying, "Hold on, Bob. Betsy has been following your advice faithfully these past few months. She's had to undergo many changes in her lifestyle, not only for her own sake, but also to please you. We know that we're doing wrong in eating these cones, and yet we both feel that she deserves it. This is sort of a celebration for us. Last Saturday I decided to paint our bedroom. Betsy felt well enough to grab a paintbrush and work alongside me for the entire day. Six hours she painted. She enjoyed the challenge and the experience, but we knew that the next day, Sunday, she would pay the consequences with pain, probably extreme pain. Bob, it never materialized. Betsy absolutely did not have any extra pain. And even today, there has not been any increase, so that's why we decided to celebrate with ice cream cones—her first one in over six months. We just wanted to share her success with you."

"Where's my ice cream cone?" Did I say that?

This success story still brings tears of joy to my eyes.

52

Hemorrhoids

Hemorrhoids are another condition in which the deficiency is not visible. However, body language can offer clues that a deficiency may exist. My first experience with this condition involved the manager of a grocery store where I worked. I had just been transferred to this store as an assistant manager, so I wasn't privy to the many jokes circulating amongst the employees about him. The jokes manifested when he had difficulty in either walking or sitting. I asked one of the grocery clerks why he wasn't involved with these stories and jokes about Mr. Russell.

"If those clerks knew what Mr. Russell was going through, they wouldn't make fun of him." He understood because for years he had suffered with this condition before ultimately having surgery. In spite of the operation, he still had great discomfort and pain.

Mr. Russell had what is called prolapsed hemorrhoids, which may cause severe rectal bleeding, pain, and lots of rectal itching. The grocery clerk explained that Mr. Russell would go behind a counter or somewhere else out of view to scratch in private.

My next experience with this health problem was years later. While standing in line at a Los Angeles Dodgers baseball game for some Dodger Dogs, I overheard two men in line behind me discussing their hemorrhoid problems and treatment. One man stated that his doctor recommended he "lasso" his swollen hemorrhoid with a rubber band and then continue wrapping the rubber band around it until it was tight enough to stay in place. Eventually, he continued, as the rubber band cut off the flow of blood to the swollen hemorrhoid, the hemorrhoid would die and fall off. They both laughed, but the friend didn't believe him. The teller of the story finally admitted that the doctor applied the rubber band with an instrument called a proctoscope, and, except for an uncomfortable feeling, it was relatively painless. He had the procedure done many times, which to me proved that this medical procedure did not correct the problem. That's when I got involved.

On a piece of paper I wrote: *From personal experience, try taking one 500 mg bioflavonoid capsule three times a day for two weeks. Then, one a day until the bottle is empty. Continue use only if problem comes back.*

I handed the note to the teller of the story and told him to get his pharmacist to fill this prescription for him. As he and his friend read the note, I purchased my Dodger Dogs. As I walked past them, I said, "This regimen worked for many of my clients."

Did he follow my suggestion? I'll never know, but if he did he would be correcting just part of the problem. Hopefully, his pharmacist would tell him to drink more water, increase his fiber intake, and, to improve his bowel movements, to take the mineral magnesium. Collectively, these steps would help correct the problem.

53

PREGNANCY AND HEMORRHOIDS

Julie, who was both a co-worker and friend of my wife, suffered from hemorrhoids. It was a condition she, and many others like her, never discussed with anyone except their doctor. In Julie's case this was unfortunate because, had she known about it, my wife could have lessened Julie's pain and suffering months earlier.

Julie's problem started during the second trimester of her first pregnancy. During this time, she and my wife worked together in a very exclusive and fashionable women's boutique. As Julie's condition worsened, her time off from work increased due to the pain. The employer asked Pat, my wife, if there was something that could be done nutritionally.

Since Julie wouldn't discuss her problem openly, Pat was in a dilemma about how to approach her. Additionally, Julie would never consider using the "H" word, especially in public, and not wanting to alienate Julie, Pat hesitated in talking to her.

One particularly busy Saturday, Pat called me saying that Julie was having a most difficult time. She couldn't walk, couldn't sit, and could hardly stand. What could I do to help her? For me this was not a problem, because I didn't mind the embarrassment. I wanted to help her lessen her painful condition.

It was easy: I went to the boutique, walked over to the hurting Julie, and handed her a bag with a bottle in it. Before she could ask what it was, I told her it was something called bioflavonoids and was for her hemorrhoids. Of course, she was embarrassed and a little upset, but I continued talking. I told her that if her doctor were aware of this product, he would tell her to take one pill immediately, another with lunch, one more at dinner, and one at bedtime, then continue with the same routine tomorrow. I told her to trust me. Then I did an about-face and left the store.

On Monday morning when Pat arrived for work, the first person she saw was Julie, who had a big grin on her face. Julie confided in Pat that she had taken the miracle drug I had given her and by Sunday afternoon could sit, walk, and even run.

Now that Julie was responsive and willing to discuss her problem with Pat and me, I scheduled an appointment for counseling. In addition to the bioflavonoids, Julie promised she would add more fiber to her diet. Additionally, she bought the mineral magnesium, a natural iron, which was not constipating, and a multivitamin.

For the next seven years that we knew Julie, not once did she ever have another episode with hemorrhoids; and, yes, they did have another child, in fact, two children—twins.

54

PMS

Although I enjoy going to the zoo, I hurt for many of the animals that are confined to their cages rather than having the entire world to run, fly, or crawl about. Especially the cats. Seeing them pace, back and forth, back and forth, in their cages, going from one end to the other only to be separated from freedom by iron bars.

Our friend Wathena reminded me of such an animal, as she paced back and forth in our living room, just like a caged tiger. "What's the matter, Wathena? You seem very edgy."

"It's that stupid time of the month. You know," she answered.

"No, I don't know. Well, I used to know, but since Pat and I got into the vitamin industry, she hasn't had that problem."

Wathena looked at my wife quizzically.

Pat nodded, saying, "I used to have that problem. We jokingly called it "premenstrual witchiness," but my daughters and I don't have the problem anymore—not since we learned about vitamin B-6."

"Talk to me," said Wathena. "But first, do you happen to have an extra B-6 pill handy? If it works, I want to take it now."

We did have some, of course, and offered one along with a glass of water.

"Maybe I should take a few more, my problem is so awful. And you're right, I do feel witchy."

We told her about our many customers who had responded positively to this vitamin. We probably had more men requesting this B-6 than women. They realized the important role this vitamin plays during a woman's menstrual cycle. Vitamin B-6 is a diuretic that lessens bloating, breast tenderness, leg cramping, and the need to cry.

As for how much to take, most customers prefer a small dosage—25 mg—but it can be taken as many as four, five, or six times a day. "It's better to take it as needed," Pat explained, "than to take one high-potency pill." She added that, in addition, a person must take a B-complex so as to not upset the balance of the B vitamins.

In less than an hour, Wathena was feeling better. A month later, after purchasing some B-6 for herself, she called to say, "The vitamin really works!" She became a true believer and never had to pace like a tiger again.

55

SLUMPED SHOULDERS

While waiting for my order at a local delicatessen, I noticed that one of the younger waitresses had very slumped shoulders. Slumped shoulders could be caused by trying to appear shorter, trying to hide excessive breast endowment, or by severe menstrual cramping.

This young waitress seemed to fall into the third category. If she had been in my store with her mother, it would have been easy to approach her. Fortunately, I knew the manager of the deli so I asked to see her. Hopefully, she would be on duty at this time.

"Hi, Bob, how can I help you?" Elsie asked.

"Elsie, how well do you know the young waitress with the ponytail?"

"Very well, she's my daughter. Why?"

"The way she's standing makes me think she has a nutritional deficiency. I've got to ask you a very personal question about her, if you don't mind."

"Bob, I didn't know you can see deficiencies of vitamins. How do you do it?"

"Anyone can do it; it just takes practice. It's okay to ask you, then?"

She nodded yes.

"Does your daughter have severe menstrual cramping?"

"Oh my gosh, does she ever. How did you know? She's on pain medication for it. She dreads having a period. What can be done?"

"Slow down, Elsie. Her slumped shoulders gave me my first clue. You just confirmed my suspicion. Does she also have difficulty falling asleep or leg cramps?"

She nodded her head yes.

"Elsie, based on your answers, your daughter is deficient in minerals. I'll bring a bottle over to you this afternoon. Do you think she would prefer a tablet or a capsule?"

Elsie settled on a capsule.

Two months or, more precisely, two menstrual cycles later, Elsie confided that her daughter's problem had lessened to the point where she no longer needed pain medication. She had waited until after the second cycle to tell me, in case it was just psychological.

Once, while I was having lunch in Sacramento, California, with my granddaughter and her husband, everyone in our party noticed the slumping of our waitress's shoulders. I told my family the story of Elsie's daughter. My granddaughter insisted we help this girl. I wrote down what she needed to buy if she had the following symptoms: leg cramping, dental problems, difficulty sleeping, and, of course, menstrual cramping. Lisa, my granddaughter, gave the note to our waitress as we left. The waitress confided in Lisa that she did have all of those problems and said she would buy a multi-mineral formula when she got off duty. Hopefully, she kept this promise.

56

Kidney Stones

As I sit here typing away on this book, I think of the many times nutrition was not allowed to play a positive role in correcting obvious deficiencies. It was always either a relative or a very close friend whom I could not convince. That's the difference between the attitudes of these friends and relatives and those of my customers. My customers seemed to trust me and at least consider my suggestions and advice. This next story illustrates what I mean.

"Bob, I owe you a four-year apology. You were right."

With that statement, my dear friend and buddy asked if I would fill the "non" prescription he had just received from his doctor. Although written on a prescription paper, it was really a reminder for my friend to purchase some magnesium and vitamin B-6.

Four years earlier my dear friend had visited me at one of my retail stores and commented that he'd had another kidney stone attack.

"Do you also have constipation?"

"No, not really."

"Let me clarify my question. Do you have, at the very least, one bowel movement daily?"

"No, I don't, but the doctor said that if I 'go' every other day on a regular basis, it's considered normal."

"If your dogs had bowel movements every other day, would you consider that normal as well?" I knew my friend loved his two dogs. When I asked that question, I knew he would answer more realistically.

"You're right. I have constipation."

"Are your teeth sensitive to hot or cold?"

"Yes, yes. What are you trying to sell me?"

"Only on an idea, not on any product."

Although my friend did take a multiple vitamin plus a little of vitamins C and E, he was more prone to listen to the medical field for nutritional advice. I suggested that he either consider including some magnesium and vitamin B-6 into his diet or, at the very least, talk to his doctor about these two supplements.

"If the doctor thought they were necessary, he would have prescribed them long ago." Period. I was excused. There would be no more discussion about his problem and/or solution.

Unfortunately, over the next four years, my friend had at least ten or more kidney stone attacks. And those were the ones I knew about. Two of the attacks required surgery, and one of them almost cost him his life. But he persisted in believing that medication alone would correct his problem. That is why the apology caught me by surprise. In a very matter-of-fact way, I just answered, "Okay." There was no need to gloat or say, "I told you so." I was just pleased that my friend was now, in my opinion, doing the right thing. Over the next several years before his death, he never had another kidney stone attack.

57

Eyes - Twitching

It is disturbing when people say that vitamins are not necessary and are a waste of money. I usually ask them why breakfast cereals are fortified with vitamins or why they are not supposed to rinse their rice before cooking? They are mildly shocked when I tell them that most cereals are dead foods, vitamin-wise, and that that's why they have to be added. Rice shouldn't be rinsed because rinsing washes off the vitamin coating that has been added.

Fortunately, my customers have both trust and faith in my industry. Without that, who knows how this next story would have ended? Perhaps with a colonectomy.

I exchanged greetings with a customer who said, "Thank you for what you did for my son twelve years ago."

What a nice way to start the day, with a very sincere thank you and a compliment as well. This customer had been buying supplements from me for twelve years. Such loyalty and trust.

Roseanne introduced me to her son, a young man dressed in army fatigues. "Bob, this is my son Matt; he's the one whose life you changed when he was just eight years old. That's why I said the thank you."

At that moment, I recalled the incident to which she was referring. As Roseanne said, it had happened twelve years earlier. It must have been on a weekday, because she came by after picking her son up from school. It was flu season and she wanted to stock up on vitamin C and a very popular and effective item for combating the flu called the Wellness Formula. Her son, as many children do when they are bored, stood at the front door waiting impatiently for his mother. That's when I noticed a continuous twitching in his right eye, so I asked her about it.

"Oh, that twitching stuff has been going on for several years now. The doctor diagnosed it as a nervous condition that was probably caused by family stress, such as a split home. That, combined with the strain associated with school, causes the eye to go into spasm."

Could be, I thought, *but it could be associated with a deficiency of a particular mineral.* I had to find out if my hunch was correct. Very discreetly, so her son could not hear, I asked Roseanne if he had at least two bowel movements a day. Direct questions like this one always catch people off guard. She smiled at first and then, whispering, said he did not. She continued, "In fact, we're lucky if he goes every third day."

I continued asking her questions. Initially, regarding his teeth.

"Are his teeth sensitive to hot or cold?"

"Yes."

"Does he have difficulty sleeping or falling asleep?"

This time it was a very resounding, "Yes."

I asked several other questions relating to specific supplements, including vitamin B-1, pantothenic acid, and calcium. My conclusion, based on the several *yes* answers, was that her son was deficient in magnesium. That's what I suggested she buy twelve years ago, and she did.

It's comforting when customers trust me, especially when my suggestions or recommendations are in opposition to those of the medical world. In this situation Roseanne, with a spirit of confidence, said to her son, "This is going to help you with your bathroom problem." And it did and still does. A life changed just because of a twitching eye.Let the twitch continue...

A customer who has now become a close friend was in the store one Saturday morning. In the middle of our conversation, I asked him if I could ask a very personal question. Somewhat shocked and perhaps amused, he answered, "Sure, why not?"

"Daniel, do you have constipation?"

He laughed aloud and asked me, "Where did that come from? I mean, here we are talking about going dancing with our wives and, out of this conversation, you ask me if I'm constipated. Where did that come from?"

"Are you?" I countered.

"Yes, but what prompted you to ask me?"

"I noticed that your eye was twitching and that's usually associated with a magnesium deficiency."

He answered with a light profanity and then laughed at me some more. "My dear friend, you're something else. Do you ask everybody if they're constipated?"

"Yes, despite any embarrassment, I do. If I can help someone who has a correctable condition, I'll ask the question."

"Bob, I have magnesium at home. You mean that if I take it my eye twitches will go away?"

"Probably, and so will your constipation, as both of them are associated with a magnesium deficiency."

On Tuesday of the next week Daniel came into the store and gave me a high five. Then he said, "Let's make it a double high five. One has stopped and the other is moving. Thanks for being so bold, I really appreciate it."

58

A Sty in the Eye

Iodine is a mineral needed by the body in trace amounts, micrograms to be exact. Its deficiency is most noticeable in people's eyes, hair, or fingernails. In this story a deficiency of this mineral was apparent, but because I knew one of the two customers quite well, I decided to play with the situation.

"Good morning, Kathy. Is this pretty young lady your sister?"

"Hi, Bob. No, this isn't my sister; she's a dear friend who is visiting me from out of state. Marcie, this is Bob, my vitamin man." Then Kathy added, "Bob, Marcie doesn't believe in vitamins."

"Is that true, Marcie?" I asked.

"Oh, I believe in vitamins, but I get enough in my diet. I live on a farm, and I get enough from the fresh foods I eat."

"Where are you from, Marcie—Illinois, Missouri, or Iowa?"

"I'm from Illinois," she answered, astonished. "But how did you know I'm from the Midwest?"

"Your eyes told me," I said matter-of-factly.

"You are kidding, aren't you?" she asked.

"No, I'm not kidding. It was your eyes. They're talking to me. Both of them."

Marcie looked over at Kathy, who was grinning.

"It's like I told you in the car, Marcie, he's learned that deficiencies are visible, and he's seeing something in your eyes."

Marcie looked back at me and asked somewhat sarcastically, "Are you saying my eyes just spelled out I-l-l-i-n-o-i-s? That's incredible!"

I agreed that they hadn't. I then told her I had noticed she was squinting. That usually means a person has eye sensitivity to light, which is associated with deficiencies of several different nutrients. I waited for her to acknowledge my statement before I continued.

"Okay, I admit to having that problem, but lots of people squint. I still don't understand how you could draw a conclusion from that."

"Marcie, I look for symptoms of a nutrient deficiency through what I call "body language." The body, your body, tells you when you have a problem. In your case, you have a probable deficiency of the mineral iodine."

I told her that squinting and sensitivity to light were the first two clues, and clue number three was seeing a sty in each of her eyes. All three clues are symptomatic of a deficiency of either vitamin A or the mineral iodine. But because she lives on a farm, the chance of a vitamin A deficiency would be remote, as most farms have gardens yielding fresh vegetables.

"Sounds very interesting, but I'm still not sure I understand what body language is."

"Marcie, do you ever have a headache?" I asked.

"Why yes, of course. Doesn't everybody at some time?"

"Yes, to answer your question. But to my way of thinking, a headache is body language in action. The body is telling you that you are at dis-ease. A toothache, a joint pain, leg cramps, menstrual cramping, and acne are additional examples of your body telling you that you have a problem."

"Couldn't those also be symptoms of a disease or illness?" asked Marcie.

Kathy jumped in, "Marcie, there is no difference, except that what doctors have to test to see Bob sees as deficiencies of nutrients." Then she added, "And I'm beginning to learn how to do it myself."

"Okay, but how did my eyes tell you I'm from the Midwest?"

"As far as which state, that was a guess. But as for your being from the Midwest, that was an educated guess based on your statement that you live on a farm. Since the Midwest is known as farm country, and deficiencies of iodine are inherent in that part of the country, it seemed logical that that was where you lived."

Marcie looked at me wide-eyed.

"You don't use iodized salt, do you?" I asked.

"No, we don't use that kind of salt. Mom used to say that iodine is something you put on wounds and it's not for eating. As for my sties, yes, I always get them, but the doctor calls them a hordeolum, an infection of some sort. You're saying that if I add iodine to my diet, I won't get them anymore? What a relief it would be to be rid of them."

Marcie grabbed my hand and, while holding it, asked in a playful and teasing way, "Are there any other body parts of mine that show deficiencies?"

"Your hair and fingernails."

"What? Do you mean they were talking to you, too?"

"Yes, Marcie. I noticed that your fingernails appear somewhat brittle and your hair is a little on the dry side—additional indications of iodine deficiency. Do you ever suffer from a stuffy nose?"

"Even my nose is talking to you? Is a stuffy nose also a sign of iodine deficiency?"

"Yes, Marcie, it is. Now you get the idea. Even a person's nose does the talking, if you know exactly what it and the rest of the body are saying. Many of the symptoms your body has displayed could be related to deficiencies of other vitamins or minerals, but the accumulation of your *yes* answers to my questions points to a deficiency of iodine."

Marcie looked at Kathy, who was grinning, and asked if she could use her cell phone. She wanted to call her mom and tell her to buy some iodized salt.

59

FINGERNAILS

Fingernails can be very revealing, both cosmetically and, especially, health-wise. I always look at a customer's fingernails, because any abnormality can indicate a diet that lacks nutrients.

Women are especially concerned about the condition of their fingernails and appreciate help in correcting problems. Sometimes they are a little embarrassed when I make them aware of an issue, but they eventually appreciate my informing them of what I see. And what do I see?

My job is easier when they're not wearing acrylics or their fingernails are polish-free, but there are ways around those two situations. If a woman is wearing acrylics, I compliment her fingernails, going on the assumption that they are real. That usually brings, "Oh, they're not real." Then I ask, "Do you have difficulty with your nails?" A *yes* generates the question, "What kind of problem?" If she is not wearing acrylics, I can see signs of deficiency and make suggestions accordingly.

Brittle fingernails prompts additional questions including, "Do you have dry hair?" (If I've already noticed that her hair is dry, I ask about or look at her fingernails for an additional clue.) "Do you have a stuffy nose?" "Are your eyes sensitive to light?" (If she's wearing sunglasses indoors, this prompts me to ask about fingernails and/or dry hair because there is a correlation). *Yes* answers to these questions indicate a deficiency of the mineral iodine, which is available in kelp tablets and by eating seafood.

If the fingernails are unpolished, I look for either longitudinal lines or a pale skin color under the nails. If these are present, I suspect anemia. I take note of the palms of the hands, the skin color of the face, and/or shortness of breath—additional recognizable symptoms of anemia.

If the nails look as if they split, are thin, or don't appear to grow, these signs indicate either a lack of protein or vitamin A or both. If the client is lacking protein, I ask about his or her protein intake. If protein intake is adequate and yet protein deficiency is the cause of the fingernail problem, then I suspect a lack of protein assimilation, which prompts questions related to a hydrochloric acid deficiency.

Hangnails usually indicate the lack of vitamin C as well as protein, whereas felons, a painful infection at the end of a finger or toe, cause me to suspect a viral infection. That prompts questions about a copper deficiency.

Again, if the fingernails are brittle, the hair dry, and the eyes sensitive to light, I start asking questions related to a thyroid condition. After several additional *yes* answers, the client usually asks what his or her problem is or says, "Wow, you really know a lot about me" or asks if I'm a doctor. The last question is the most laughable, as so few doctors know the visible or tactile symptoms related to a thyroid condition. Doctors rely on a series of blood tests to determine these conditions. However, if a doctor was to greet his or her new patient with a handshake, he or she could determine just by touching the patient's hand that the person might have a thyroid condition, blood sugar condition, or other condition, including Raynaud's disease. Simply by touching someone's hand.

Once I have established that my client might have a thyroid deficiency, I ask questions related to a deficiency of vitamin A. I usually get several *yes* answers about that as well. With all of these *yeses*, is it any wonder that these people are also tired, overweight, constipated, catch cold easily, suffer from sinus problems and even diminished libido? Just by looking at their fingernails and asking questions I can usually find the root cause or symptoms of many disorders.

If the fingernails are brittle, I suspect an iodine deficiency and ask questions accordingly. If I get additional *yeses*, I ask about their thyroid gland and vitamin A. If the fingernails are brittle and they are not wearing acrylics, I look for the natural color of the fingernail. If these are too light or white, I ask questions related to an iron deficiency. Brittle fingernails can also indicate a total lack of minerals, or if there are sufficient minerals in the diet, a lack of hydrochloric acid. Brittleness can also indicate a lack of protein, or if there is sufficient protein in the diet, again, a lack of hydrochloric acid.

60

Dry Hair

A very professional-appearing young woman, probably in her late twenties, wanted to know about the Body Language Questionnaire I offer to my customers. I gave her a copy and explained to her how it works.

"Can I complete it now?" she asked.

"Of course."

As she started to scrutinize the questionnaire, I noticed that her hair was very dry, too dry. "Thyroid or too much hair dye?" I wondered. I made a mental note to check the sections on the questionnaire pertaining to thyroid. I looked at her fingernails for an additional clue, but she was wearing acrylics so I couldn't see any signs in her nails. Her eyes. Did the bright lights seem to bother her? Was she squinting? Her next comment broke into my thoughts.

"I certainly didn't enter very many check marks; in fact, I only answered four. Four out of, let's see, two hundred and eighty questions. Not bad."

Usually, it's the men who don't answer all the questions that pertain to them. In this case, this young woman, who had, at the least, four noticeable deficiencies, decided not to be honest with herself.

I quickly looked over the questionnaire to determine to what areas the four check marks applied. The thyroid, vitamin B-12, pantothenic acid, and iodine sections were marked, but I also noticed there were about ten boxes that had been marked and then erased. Those areas were: enzymes, vitamin A, most of the B vitamins, and hydrochloric acid. I started with asking questions relevant to iodine.

"You marked that you have a problem with your fingernails. What kind of problem?"

"They're brittle, dry, and they split."

"What about your hair? Isn't it slightly dry, too?"

"Yes. I guess slightly. Anyway, my beautician is helping me with that problem, so I didn't mark that box."

Two of the erasures were in the iodine section, so I suggested that iodine, or kelp tablets, should be on her purchase list.

"Thank you, but before I buy iodine, I'm going to check with my beautician first."

Okay, I thought, then continued. "Enzymes. I noticed that you had marked four boxes *yes* and then erased the marks. What are they? *Yeses* or *nos*?"

"They're both, but not all the time. Only when I eat crazily."

"Based on the number of *yeses* for enzymes, you should consider taking them, if only for the times you eat crazily. They help assimilate whatever food you eat."

"Ah, I think I'll check with my friend about that item, too."

"You're lacking vitamin B-12. Although you only marked that area one time, you had three erasures. This vitamin could be another cause of the excessive dryness of your fingernails."

"That's interesting. I have to check with my beautician about a lot. Before I buy anything, I mean."

Okay, I thought, *maybe her beautician is also a nutritionist or certainly aware of nutrition.* So I asked her, "Is your beautician a nutritionist?"

"No, but she knows a lot about health."

I wondered if her reluctance to buy was due to a lack of money. I didn't ask her, but instead continued with the evaluation.

"Your fingernails, besides being both dry and brittle, have ridges that seem to be going both up and down across the nails. This could indicate a lack of the entire family of B vitamins. Do you currently take a B-complex or a multiple vitamin?"

"No."

"It's also a good idea to start with the basics. Perhaps a multiple vitamin is better because it contains vitamin A, which is also a fingernail vitamin."

"Oh, I'm not sure I need a multiple. I had better check with my beautician first."

"Susan," I read her name from the questionnaire. "You keep telling me that you have to check with your beautician first before you make any purchases. Is it because you don't trust my judgment or is there some other reason you're not buying—a lack of funds, perhaps?"

"Oh no, I have the money. I have a good-paying job, and it's certainly not you. It's because of your reputation that I'm in here. It's just that she knows so much about health problems and I want to ask her opinion before I buy anything."

"Well, Susan, I can certainly appreciate that. Tell me, did your beautician make you aware of any of these deficiencies we've been discussing? Specifically the enzymes, B-12, iodine, and the B-complex vitamins, and that they might be the cause of your fingernail problems?"

She answered no.

I continued. "Susan, I would like to conduct a seminar at your friend's place of business. She could invite her customers, friends, and, of course, her employees. Would you like to ask her about inviting me?"

"Oh, that would be great. Would you talk about nutrition?"

"No. I want to talk to the group about cosmetics and hair sprays and hair dryers, and things like that."

"What do you know about those things?"

"Susan, I know as much about your friend's industry as she knows about mine." I said with a slight grin.

Her eyes started to well up with tears. "Oh, I am so sorry. I didn't mean to doubt you, and I don't, it's just that, that, oh, I am so sorry. You have spent so much of your time with me and I didn't even appreciate it. You are right, I mean, you do know a lot, a lot more than my friend. I came here for help, you offered me help, and I didn't accept it. I am sorry."

"Susan, maybe you could talk to your friend about my doing a lecture on nutrition at her place of business. What do you think?"

Susan heeded my advice, and over the next few months most of her conditions were corrected. No, I never did give the lecture at her beautician's place of business, but she too became a customer of mine and began handing out our Body Language Questionnaire to her clients who had problems similar to Susan's.

61

Trembling Hands and Fingers

One of the perils of owning a retail store is having a customer's check returned from the bank as un-depositable funds. Upon picking up my mail from the post office, I saw an ominous envelope from my bank. Inside was a check from one of my regular customers that had been returned because of an unauthorized signature. Technically, that means the signature was forged. I telephoned the customer to make him aware of his returned check.

"I'll be right over and make it right to you," the customer responded.

I welcomed his willingness to correct the problem, but I wondered why he would make a check good if it was forged. I pondered this question until he arrived a couple of hours later.

"Hey, Sam, thanks for your quick response in this matter."

"Hi, Bob. I'm so sorry for this inconvenience, which is all my fault. I just came from the bank and explained to them my signature inconsistency. I'll write out a new check for you, if you don't mind, or would you prefer cash? The bank said they'll reimburse you for the check return fee."

"Sam, your check is always welcome," I was curious about the inconsistency of his signature. When he started writing out his check, I saw what he meant. His hand and fingers were trembling so badly that he could barely hold the pen.

"Hold on, Sam. I'll write the check, and you can sign it."

He thanked me and handed me his check. As I was writing, I asked what caused his trembling.

"I don't know. The doctors don't know, either. They're running different tests on me, but so far to no avail. I can't even go to work."

"When did the trembling start?"

"About three weeks ago. First, I began vomiting, and then the diarrhea started. Actually, the diarrhea was sort of a good thing as I have always been constipated, but then it wouldn't stop. We thought I just had a flu bug, and

I was treated accordingly. Within a week I was feeling better. That's when the trembling started."

I looked at Sam's eyes. His left eye was twitching.

"Sam, are you able to ride in a boat without getting sick?"

"No. I like to fish, but only from the shore. Bob, why did you ask that?"

I didn't answer, but asked another question. This time it was whether he ever experienced car sickness. Another *yes.*

"Sam, while you had the stomach flu and were vomiting and having diarrhea, how severe was the vomiting? Was it once or twice a day, or was it all the time?"

"Bob, I had to carry a plastic bag with me, the vomiting was so bad. With the diarrhea, I had to be near a bathroom at all times. My doctor said I had one of the worst cases of the flu he had ever treated."

"Sam, before I fill in the amount of this check, I would like to add to the total."

"What for? Just because you wrote the check for me?" he asked with a grin.

"No, I want to include the cost of some vitamin B-6 and magnesium. I have a hunch, based on your answers, that you developed a deficiency of these two items during your severe episode of vomiting and diarrhea."

Sam returned to work the following week.

62

Prolapsed Colon

What do you say first to a woman you suspect has a prolapsed colon, constipation, frequent urination, and probably a tipped uterus? How about, "Excuse me ma'am, but do you happen to have a problem with your intestines?" Now, I ask people embarrassing questions regarding their obvious nutritional deficiencies, but in this situation I felt stymied. So I said, "Good morning, how may I help you?"

"Oh, I'm just looking." Her answer was unhelpful.

When I receive this answer, I wait a few minutes and approach the customer with the following: "What are you looking for? Perhaps I can help you find it."

"Oh, thank you, but I'm just looking."

Still no help.

"Ma'am, we have several items on sale including vitamin E, magnesium, and psyllium powder, which is also referred to as colon cleanse." I had just committed a peccadillo because the psyllium powder wasn't really on sale, but I needed to include it in the list.

"What's psyllium powder?" she asked.

"It's useful in promoting a bowel movement. Do you know of anyone who has a problem with constipation?" By asking her if she knew someone else, I wouldn't be embarrassing her if she was the one with the problem.

"That product certainly isn't for me then. I am very regular."

Ouch. There went my theory. But I wasn't satisfied with her answer, and so I pushed for a clarification as to what "very regular" meant to her.

"Oh, you're one of the lucky ones who have at least two bowel movements every day."

"Who said I had two bowel movements a day?"

I was correct after all. I continued, "If not two a day, does that mean three or just one?" I was forcing her to give a definite number.

"I have a bowel movement every fourth day." She almost beamed with pride as she answered my question. "And, according to my doctor, so long as I'm consistent, regular every fourth day, I'm not constipated." She was still beaming.

During our brief conversation, I had picked up a container of psyllium powder. I handed it to her. This enabled me to get within inches of her and do the sniff test. Again, I had to confirm another suspicion.

Sniff test, frequent urination, prolapsed colon. You might be asking what I saw that led me to conclude that she might have these problems? First, she was overweight, but that's common nowadays. Second, her stomach was literally sagging and several inches below the belt. Third, she was perspiring on a rather chilly morning. Conclusion? I suspected a prolapsed colon.

How did I reach that conclusion, and what is a prolapsed colon? The colon is a tube a little less than five feet long, located in the abdomen and shaped like an irregular square. At its start, it's linked to the small intestine, or ileum, at a juncture called the cecum or ileocecal valve. From there, the colon extends upward toward the liver to what is known as the hepatic flexure. Then it transverses left across the abdomen, toward the spleen, where it is attached to the splenic flexure. From this point, the colon bends downward and descends to the Sigmoid colon, ending at the anus. When the colon is exceptionally full of fecal matter that cannot be eliminated, the weight will occasionally cause the transverse portion of the colon to drop or prolapse. There are times when either the splenic or hepatic flexures becomes detached, causing the colon to drop. My client's stomach was drooping over her belt, and from what she had told me I knew she was chronically constipated. I concluded that a prolapsed colon might be the cause.

A prolapsed colon exerts pressure on those organs below it, specifically the uterus and bladder. If enough pressure is put on the uterus it can tip, or incline backward rather than forward. A tipped uterus is considered harmless, unless undue pressure on the bladder induces frequent urination.

If fecal matter is not being excreted adequately through timely bowel movements, the toxins within the colon are then reabsorbed into the bloodstream for elimination elsewhere in the body, sometimes through the breath, most often through the skin. At times, a slight odor emanates from the skin—thus the sniff test.

Her perspiring could be caused by many factors, including the weather, blood sugar problems, pre- or peri-menopause, or, in this instance, constipation.

Now that I had removed the embarrassment factor, we talked at great length about her various medical problems. As to the uterus, she said that hers was in a "first-degree" prolapsed state. Yes, she did have a bladder condition and was being treated for incontinence, with drugs of course. She was using mouthwash for her bad breath and a special antibacterial soap to help correct her body odor. She said that she had to shower at least twice a day to keep the odor in check.

Her answers to the Body Language Questionnaire showed me that she was deficient in magnesium, which she bought. She also bought psyllium powder, a "green" protein drink, liquid chlorophyll, and a multiple vitamin. She found a chiropractor who did what is called high enemas or colonics and, at the chiropractor's suggestion, applied warm mineral oil packs to her belly. This, along with the magnesium and chlorophyll, corrected her problem with constipation within two weeks, which thus lessened her body odor and bad breath.

Now I know what to say to a woman with a prolapsed colon.

63

Bruxism - The Grinding of Teeth

The grinding of his teeth sounded like fingernails scratching a blackboard. The perpetrator was being helped by one of my employees at the checkout counter, so I sauntered over to check out his purchase. He wasn't buying anything that would help him stop grinding his teeth. I didn't know whether my employee had suggested anything for this problem, and if she had not I didn't want to embarrass her about it so, for everyone's sake, I used caution.

I walked up to the customer and said, "Good afternoon, and thank you for your purchase."

My employee introduced us. The man's name was Stu, but his nickname was Coffee. We shook hands.

"Coffee, that's a very interesting nickname. Is it because you drink so much of it?" After asking the question, I realized how dumb it sounded.

"No, it's because I grind my teeth. My co-workers gave me that name almost ten years ago; they said I sound like a coffee grinder. It bugs them, but I can't help it. I've tried everything."

"Most everything," I said, correcting him gently. "I said 'most everything' because I believe that something causes it to happen and, if so, there is a way to correct it."

"Naw, I've tried the natural route, too. A local homeopathic doctor put me on belladonna. I tried different potencies and even varied the dosage, but it still didn't work."

"Do you also have TMJ?"

"No, I don't think so. What's that?"

"*TMJ* stands for temporomandibular joint syndrome. It usually causes extreme pain when chewing."

"No, I don't have that, but maybe the splint the dentist put on me is helping."

"Is there a family history of blood sugar problems like hypoglycemia, diabetes, or even alcoholism?"

"Yes, Mom and Dad both have diabetes. Dad used to drink a lot. Why do you ask?"

To maintain my train of thought I usually answer a question with a question. I asked him if he had a drinking problem. He answered no, but did answer yes to my next question about eating lots of sweets, particularly ice cream or candy.

"Do you have about fifteen minutes to answer some questions on this Body Language Questionnaire? Specifically, those sections I have marked?"

"Why do you want me to do this? Why did you ask me about sugar problems?"

I explained that, when we shook hands, I noticed his palms were moist. That could indicate a pancreatic or adrenal problem or both. Answering the questions in the sections I marked would help me determine what might make him grind his teeth.

Reluctantly, Stu completed the sections I had asked him to answer and then handed me the paper. "Interesting questions. I've never been asked them before, not even with the homeopathic doctor. She said to take the belladonna. Okay, what's wrong, or do I have to come back for the answers?"

I read over the questionnaire and found, based on his answers, that he was probably deficient in calcium, magnesium, potassium, chromium, and pantothenic acid and that he might have a tendency toward hypoglycemia. The questionnaire does not reveal diseases as such, but it does indicate weaknesses in the body that correlate to some illnesses. With both of his parents being alcoholic, hypoglycemia in an offspring is almost a given.

"What kind of work do you do, Stu?"

"Heavy construction."

"Do you take salt pills when the weather is this hot?"

He said he did take them and sometimes took as many as ten to twenty pills a day. He added that he needed to because he sweats a lot. "Almost like a continuous stream of water," he added, laughing.

At the beginning of this conversation he was grinding his teeth, but only slightly. As my questioning became more personal, the intensity of the grinding increased. I was obviously stressing him. In many cases, stress is one of the causes of bruxism. Additionally, all the nutrients that he was apparently deficient in were indicated to correct this condition.

Sometimes chromium is indicated for those who are afflicted with low blood sugar. Calcium and magnesium have both been determined to help in correcting bruxism. Pantothenic acid, which helps in reducing the stress, was also indicated. He said he suffered from headaches as well as dizziness upon arising, which are additional symptoms of a deficiency of this vitamin.

I recommended that he see his doctor for a blood test to determine his mineral balance, specifically his potassium-to-sodium ratio. I believed he was extremely deficient in potassium. He answered that he had very little energy, suffered from a dry mouth, craved bananas, and took copious amounts of salt.

I also suggested that he complete the questionnaire at home and bring it back along with the results from his doctor. He asked me about the questionnaire my employee had already put in his bag along with the supplements he had bought from her.

"It's for someone you love," my employee said.

About two weeks later, Stu returned with his completed questionnaire in hand. I told him I would computerize it and have the results the next day. I asked if he could return then for counseling. He said Saturday would be better. He added that his doctor had told him to stop taking so many salt pills as they "could disrupt his sodium-to-potassium ratio."

On Saturday, Stu and I reviewed his questionnaire and the results of his blood test. He had such an extreme excess of sodium that the doctor prescribed a potassium supplement much higher in potency than what we offered. He did purchase the minerals that were indicated and then bade me farewell.

He called a month later and said his teeth grinding had diminished significantly. Although his doctor didn't recognize hypoglycemia as a disease, Stu decided to adopt a diet that was high in protein and low in carbohydrates. His energy level was back to normal, headaches were rare, and the dizziness was gone completely. He knew that, in time and with a continuation of supplements and diet, his bruxism would be totally corrected.

64

Toenails - Fungal Infection

It's not very often you get to see another man's toenails, unless he wears toeless shoes or goes barefoot. My friend and brother-in-law, Gerald, neither wore sandals nor went barefoot. That's why it took over forty years before I saw his condition—a fungal infection on both of his big toes.

We were both at a family reunion in Memphis and staying at the same hotel. I had gone to Gerald's room to confirm the time we were to have dinner. When he opened the door I noticed that he was barefoot, and so I made the comment, "Oh, my goodness, Gerald has feet."

He laughed and asked if I would kiss them and make them better, then lifted one leg so I could get a closer look at his foot. I quickly realized what his comment meant.

His toe was covered with a fungus that had permeated both the underside and the edges of his nail. It certainly looked gross. "That's why I always wear white socks, even when it's not stylish," he said. He showed me the other foot, and its big toe's nail was just as bad. "Son, what can you do for me? Is there a vitamin that can heal this? The doctors haven't been able to, but, then again, I'm not the best of patients either."

He had suffered from this problem since World War II when he was an infantryman in the Pacific. "It rained every day and every night, and when it didn't rain we were walking and even sleeping in water or mud. It was impossible to dry out our socks. When we tried to hang them up in the sun we were attacked, either by the enemy or by the mosquitoes. And, son, you don't get very far in the jungle running barefoot. After the war, I went to the army hospital for both my malaria and my toes, but I'm still suffering. Son, the war's not over for me—I've been suffering over fifty years of hell. The only reason I don't complain is that some of my war buddies suffer even more."

Within two weeks, Gerald's condition had improved dramatically. The results could have been even better, but, as he said, he wasn't the best of patients. Gerald used GSE (grapefruit seed extract) topically. It was difficult to convince him, a "real soldier," to dilute the GSE according to directions, but after awhile he did listen. He broke open capsules of acidophilus and applied the powder directly to his toes, and then carefully slipped into his, yes, white socks. He also took acidophilus orally.

Gerald also looked up a couple of his army buddies who had been with him in the Pacific Islands and told them that they, too, could be helped. Then he told them what he had done and how his toenails were almost normal again, after fifty years.

65

YAWNING

Just looking at the word *yawn* makes me want to yawn. Does it affect you the same way?

One could easily see that the young girl did not want to be with her mother, shopping for vitamins. She slumped against the doorframe, waiting impatiently. I guessed her age to be fourteen. She was obviously bored and, according to her posture and continuous yawning, extremely tired.

"Hurry up, Mom. I'm tired. I want to go home. Can I wait for you in the car?"

"Honey, I'm almost through and, no, you cannot wait in the car. It's too hot outside. You'd burn up in the car."

Again the young girl yawned and rubbed her eyes.

"Honey, bring me my purse," the mother said as she sidled up to the check-out counter. I, too, walked to the checkstand, even though I was not the one waiting on her. I had to check out the girl's hands, fingernails, and hair. Yes, I was looking for clues as to why she was so tired.

Her hair looked just fine, but her fingernails, although otherwise normal, were very pale. As she handed the purse to her mother, I was able to look at the palm of her hand. It, too, was very pale.

"What can I do for my daughter? She's always so tired. The doctor said it was just too much school activity, but it doesn't seem normal to me. Any suggestions?"

My employee handed her a Body Language Questionnaire and explained its function. The mother was very impressed with the few questions she read.

"Mom, if it's homework, I'm not going to do it. I have enough homework already."

The mother could answer most of the questions for her daughter. At least we could get a reasonable idea of what the problem might be.

Now I joined the conversation. "Has your daughter started her menstruating cycle yet?" I asked. Both mother and daughter looked at me—the daughter with embarrassment, the mother with surprise. Before either could answer, I continued my questioning.

"I noticed that your daughter was doing a lot of yawning. This could indicate that she's tired, of course, but it could also mean that her body is trying to increase her blood oxygen level. It's an involuntary action. I also noticed that her fingernails and palms are rather pale. These together could indicate a low iron level; that's why I asked if she has started her menstrual cycle."

The daughter was about to walk—no, run—out of the store because she was so embarrassed. "Mother, it's none of his business. Don't answer him about my personal life!" she said, almost screaming.

"Stephanie, stop right now. You're embarrassed because no one has ever asked these questions before." The mother then turned to me. "Yes, she experienced her first period two months ago."

"Since then, has she had another period and, if so, was it extremely heavy or light?" I asked.

"Yes, again on both questions, I mean, it was extremely heavy."

Stephanie walked up to the checkstand and apologized to me. "I'm sorry. I'm not used to talking to a man about these personal things, especially with you not being a doctor."

"Or a pastor," I quipped. It was enough of a little joke to cause everyone to smile.

"Did you want to ask me any other questions?"

"I want you to pull your lower eyelid down so your mother can determine the degree of redness under your lid."

"Why is that important?" she asked, but with an attitude of wonder rather than challenge. Without waiting for me to answer she pulled an eyelid down for all to see.

"It's so pale," remarked her mother. "Is that another sign of low iron?"

"Yes, it could be," I said. Then I looked at Stephanie and asked her if she ever saw spots before her eyes.

"Oh, my gosh, Mom. I've never told you because I thought I had a brain tumor or something. Yes. Yes, I do have spots before my eyes. Is that also a sign of no iron?"

I suggested that they make an appointment with their doctor and have her iron levels checked through a blood test. Meanwhile, if she would like to purchase some natural iron pills it would be okay, based on the answers I had been told.

A few weeks later, I was informed that Stephanie was doing well, and most of her symptoms of iron deficiency were gone. Surprisingly, the doctor suggested that Stephanie continue with the iron supplement I had sold her.

As I said, reading the word *yawn* makes me want to yawn, too.

66

TENDONITIS

He was a behemoth who literally filled my doorway with his mammoth body, and yet, as mammoth as he was, he appeared to be in pain. I soon found out why.

"Hey, Bob, glad you're here."

I walked over to where he was standing and extended my hand. I prepared myself for his inevitable crunching of my hand. With a certain amount of trepidation, I placed my hand into his grasp. I have a rather strong grip, but this guy was once Mr. Olympiad, Mr. World, and Mr. Universe. So I squeezed first and expected to hear the crunching of the bones, the bones in my hand.

"Ow!"

Ow? It wasn't I who said that. I started to look around to see who had said it when Steve, the gargantuan bodybuilder, continued. "Don't squeeze so hard. You're hurting my hand."

As I slacked off of my grip, I realized he had not even given me a firm handshake. Tendonitis?"

"Yes, how did you know?"

"What are you doing for it?"

"Nothing, really. The doc said it'll take time, and time I don't have. I'm supposed to compete next month, and I can't even lift twenty pounds. I guess I'll have to withdraw from competition."

"Manganese."

"Magnesium?"

"No. Manganese. It is the only mineral I'm aware of that is specifically indicated for tendonitis by Paavo Airola in his book *How to Get Well.*"

I walked over to the mineral section and picked up a bottle of manganese, 50 mg.

"Here, Steve. A doctor from New York recommended this to one of my customers for her tendonitis. He told her to take one pill three times a day."

"That many?"

"Yes. And she weighed around one hundred twenty pounds—about one-third of your body weight," I said a little sarcastically.

"Okay, you made your point. Three a day, huh? How will I know that it's working?"

"You'll know the next time you come into my store. At least, that's when I'll know."

"I don't understand. What do you mean?"

"Steve, I just whipped you badly when I shook your hand. Little me. I believe that when your hand is better, you'll want to retaliate and crunch mine. See you in about three or four weeks."

Steve did come back in four weeks, but I hesitated to shake hands with him. He was, indeed, back for vengeance. His arm was healed to the point that, two weeks later, he was well enough to compete.

Manganese has been used successfully in the treatment of allergies. Over the years, I have had several customers whose allergies have been extremely difficulty to correct. As a last resort and based on the Body Language Questionnaire, I suggested manganese, and in every case it was the determining factor in resolving their problem.

67

Broken Bones

One day in mid-September a woman in her forties came into the store. She had a cast on her leg from her hip down to her ankle; this condition required the use of crutches.

"How about a foot race?" I asked her.

She retorted, "Only if it's downhill, with the wind at my back, and I get a head start."

I liked her attitude. In spite of her obvious hurting, she maintained an upbeat demeanor. I was sure I could help her in some way, so I continued with a little bit of teasing. What I was about to learn surprised me.

"Hey, you'd better heal fast. The skiing season is just a few months away," I quipped.

This time her answer wasn't so upbeat. "Not for me, it isn't. I don't know if I'll ever be on skis again. This break appears to be forever."

Forever, I thought, *now that's a long time.* I didn't know what her condition was under the cast, but it was encouraging to hear her say it was a break. I didn't understand the "forever" part of her statement. This prompted many more questions.

The break had occurred while she was skiing at California's beautiful Mammoth Mountain the previous December. This was September, almost ten months later. According to her doctor she was not healing because of her age, which included the onset of both menopause and osteoporosis. Because of these conditions, her bones were unable to knit. She had already had several operations and was due for another in six weeks. A "telling" operation, she called it—one that could determine if she would ski again or even ever be able to walk without using some physical support. I asked her what her needs were, and she said she just needed some Echinacea for her runny nose. Her allergies seemed to be getting worse. Echinacea costs around eight or nine dollars a bottle. She left the store spending almost a hundred dollars. It was not overkill. It was the result of my asking her many of the questions found on the Body Language Questionnaire.

Her runny nose was another clue, in addition to the cast, of course. To me, it meant weak adrenal glands caused by the amount of stress she was undergoing. I pursued that hunch first with appropriate questioning that determined she needed pantothenic acid and lots of it. She was taking a multiple vitamin, but only occasionally, and promised she would definitely increase her intake to at least twice a day. As she talked, I noticed her tongue seemed to interfere with her ability to speak clearly. I asked about her thyroid, her blood pressure, and her sodium intake. She said that her blood pressure was low, but that her thyroid gland was normal. Usually low blood pressure goes hand in hand with a low thyroid, so I pursued the thyroid questions further.

Her body temperature was 98.6. That's normal. She didn't have cold hands or feet, and her heart rate was normal. One could conclude that her thyroid gland was functioning normally.

Because her doctor had said it was a good idea to restrict salt, she had put herself on a low-sodium diet. A low sodium intake combined with stressed-out adrenal glands exasperated her sodium-to-potassium ratio. She needed to increase the amount of sodium she was getting. She could do it through her diet, which would increase her energy and correct what she called her "thick tongue." Potassium is usually indicated at the onset of a stressful condition and sodium once the adrenal glands become exhausted.

Her inability to heal was due to an imbalanced diet. She was consuming too many starches and not enough protein. Her protein requirement would appear to be lessened because of her immobility, but, because of her immobility and the stress on her bones, she actually needed to increase the usual ratio of one gram to 2.2 pounds of body weight. This called for a protein supplement, and what could be better than a protein drink that included powdered lecithin and flax oil? To not lessen the normal intake of food, this drink was to be consumed after each meal as well as at bedtime along with her multiple mineral supplement. She needed the extra minerals, especially the increased calcium and magnesium that most multiple vitamins do not contain. She also purchased a combination A and D supplement, extra vitamin E, some bromelain, and the knitting herb combination called Bone, Flesh, and Cartilage. This combination of supplements should also slow down the osteoporosis. The minerals, E, and oil should help with her menopause.

I want to emphasize that the supplements she purchased would, hopefully, fill any deficiencies her body may have had, and, when they did, this should enable her body to heal itself.

Within five weeks, one week before the impending operation, she came into the store. I should say walked, minus the crutches and with the use of one cane, into the store. She was beaming from ear to ear and was equally proud to show that she was out of her hip-to-ankle cast. Much to the chagrin of her doctor, she had postponed the operation for another six weeks to see if the sudden improvement would continue.

She called me about five weeks later and said her body was continuing its healing process. The operation was subsequently cancelled, as was the need for a cane. Within six months, in February to be exact, she was skiing once again, although just on the bunny slopes. This was with the approval of her new doctor.

68

Fractured Arm

When Gary came into the store one afternoon, I had to ask him why the cast, which went from his left shoulder down to and including his wrist. He looked both pained and troubled.

"I was in a fight and obviously lost," he answered. "My brother's ex-wife was angry with him and had two of her friends go to his house with the intention of beating him up. I arrived a few minutes later and tried to help. That's when one of the guys took a swing at me with a baseball bat. I put up my arm in self-defense. He shattered the arm bones into pieces. When I fell to the ground screaming, they realized what they had done to me and took off. My brother called an ambulance and the police. According to the doctor, my arm isn't repairable. In fact, he's recommending I have it amputated and be fitted for a prosthesis."

All I could think of, besides poor Gary, was don't go near this one, Bob; it's out of your league. But I could still ask him some questions without getting involved. I started with, "How can I help?"

"Oh, Bob, I'm not expecting you to help; that's not why I came in here. I just need something for my nerves. I've got plenty of pain pills, but I want something natural for my stress. I'm going to see another doctor tomorrow for his opinion about my arm. I don't want to lose it, but the X ray doesn't look good. Again, he's pushing that I get a prosthesis instead of this dangling bunch of bones and skin."

The anguish in his eyes caused me to pursue what I have been doing since I have been in this industry—try to help in any way I can. And so I asked him, "Gary, would you mind asking your new doctor if you could take some supplements, that is, if he can save your arm?"

"What kind of vitamins are we talking about?"

First, we would have to complete a Body Language Questionnaire. I handed one to him and gave him the option of completing it there or taking it home. He chose to complete the questionnaire while I assisted other customers.

I told him about BF&C, or Bone, Flesh, and Cartilage, an herbal combination that is touted to help in the knitting of bones. And, of course, there is pantothenic acid, lots of minerals, protein, the B-complex, vitamin C, and... That's when he interrupted me.

"I want to save my arm. Do you think these things will help, even a little? I don't care what they cost, and I know that you will only sell me what I need. Please, is there hope?"

"Gary, if you're willing, I can start you on a program in concert with what your new doctor will be doing and with his approval. That is, if he thinks he can help you."

"With or without his approval, I want to get started right now. Maybe I'll see results by tomorrow."

With Gary's newfound enthusiasm, he was getting positive results already. The mind is most powerful, and he was starting to believe that his arm could be saved. Fortunately, the new doctor agreed to see what would happened with the supplements.

It has been more than four years since Gary came into the store to buy something for stress and instead bought something to save his arm. To this day, he has about 95 percent usage of his arm and wrist. He says that, once he has 100 percent usage, he wants to punch the doctor who wanted him to get a prosthesis. He was joking, of course.

69

Pain - Transitory

I had never met or talked to Candy until she called me late one Tuesday afternoon. She was crying. Through her tears she told me that she had received her completed Body Language Questionnaire from her co-worker, who had asked if he could deliver it to her. Based on what she had read on her answer sheet, something was terribly wrong with her.

"Candy, I'm sorry, but I only recognize your name. I don't recall what your results were on the profile. I don't keep a copy, so allow me to ask you a few questions; perhaps we can accomplish something on this phone call. The first thing I need to know is what are your primary problems?"

Candy told me she had been suffering for the last several months with an undiagnosed illness called migrant or transitory pain. Initially, the pain might emanate from her right ankle, go to her left knee, up to her left shoulder or arm, down to her hip, then her back, and then perhaps start all over again. The pain was almost ceaseless, continuing throughout the day and night. Yes, she was seeing a doctor; in fact, she had seen six different doctors during the previous eight months. She was currently going to the medical center of an internationally renowned university in California. They recommended that she be institutionalized until they could determine the cause of her problem.

I asked Candy a series of other questions including her age, her weight, and whether she had any children. Since she had children, I asked how long it had been since her last pregnancy and had the pregnancy been associated with any problems including third-trimester leg cramps. Candy was thirty-three, her weight was normal, she had three children—the youngest being one and a half years old. Yes, she was bedridden her last month of the pregnancy and had had severe leg cramps and toxemia.

"Bob, may my mother and I see you on Friday at eleven o'clock? Is there anything you can suggest now, over the phone? I'm so tired of hurting, and I don't want to live in a sanitarium," she said in a pleading voice.

"Candy, I'm going to tell you to do something. Please just do it and don't question me. Please." I waited for her to answer.

I could hear apprehension in her voice, perhaps even doubt about me, but she agreed to follow my recommendation.

"Go to the grocery store and buy some Gatorade. I've never tasted it, and I don't fully know why I'm suggesting it except that I have a hunch about your problem. Just do it, and we'll talk about it on Friday."

Again, with apprehension in her voice, Candy agreed.

Friday finally came, and at eleven o'clock sharp Candy walked in with her mother.

After introductions, I asked to see her profile answer sheet.

"Wait, Bob, before we do that, why did you tell me to drink Gatorade?" Candy was smiling slightly.

"I just had a suspicion about something, and that's the only thing I could think of for you to take. Okay, first, let's talk about the Gatorade. I can see in your eyes that's what you want to talk about."

Still smiling, Candy said, "After our phone conversation, I decided I would try it. After all, what did I have to lose? Well, I slept that night, almost the whole night with very little pain. Wednesday night? All sleep and no pain. And Thursday..."

Her mother chimed in at that point, not allowing Candy to finish. "Look at her, Bob, look at her. She's standing erect for the first time in months." Her mother was crying. She repeated herself. "She's standing up straight; I can't believe it."

We were all crying at that time. I guess crying can become contagious. Two of my customers and my daughter Cathy were also crying.

"Bob, why Gatorade? What made that drink work so well?" asked Candy between sobs.

"Based on your answers, my guess was that your body was trying to tell you that you had an electrolyte imbalance. That's why you had transitory pain. Leg cramps and toxemia are signals from the body that it is at dis-ease. The body is amazing, isn't it?"

"If only I had known you when I was pregnant, I probably wouldn't have suffered so much. In fact, my whole family, especially my husband, wouldn't have suffered either. Okay, I know that Gatorade was only the start. What do we do now to make sure that I'm completely well and stay that way? My husband and

I are supposed to go on a business/pleasure trip next week, and I wasn't sure I could go until yesterday—when I knew I was finally getting better."

Candy's profile answer sheet confirmed my suspicions. She was deficient in most minerals, including potassium and magnesium. Based on the results of the profile, I put her on several items. After the crying had finally stopped, and after a round of hugs, Candy and her mother left. She did call after her one-week vacation to say she never had another episode of pain. In fact, over the next several years that we kept in touch, she had no further pain.

Candy learned to listen, not only to her body but to the bodies of her children as well. She learned to determine body signals to adjust the diet or to purchase supplements to correct the problem.

One year later, against the suggestion of her doctor, Candy gave her young son a combination of cod liver oil and pantothenic acid for an ear problem. She opted for the supplements instead of the tubes that were prescribed. Yes, the nutritional combination worked.

70

Pregnancy and Calcium

The pharmaceutical company where I worked before entering the nutritional field sold one of the most popular calcium products available at that time. As an outside sales representative, it was my job to promote this product to the medical profession, with emphasis on convincing obstetricians of its effectiveness in treating third-trimester leg cramps in pregnant women. I learned from both doctors and nurses that it was effective. The nurses reported that their pregnant patients had suffered with terrible leg cramps during those last three months of pregnancy. They thanked me time and again for convincing the doctors to prescribe this mineral supplement during this important time of the pregnancy. It was obvious that these experiences would have a favorable effect on the vitamin industry.

I learned to be careful and considerate in asking questions of women regarding their possible pregnancy. However, because I had learned in the pharmaceutical industry that not many doctors were prescribing a mineral supplement to their pregnant patients, I continued my quest to inform.

After entering this industry, I learned an important lesson. Never mention pregnancy to a woman unless she mentions it first. Once I asked a woman when she was due to have her baby and was embarrassed to find out that she wasn't pregnant. Another time (I knew she was pregnant), I asked when the baby was due. She responded, in a very fractious way, that the baby had been born a month before. "Why, do I still look pregnant?"

The body tells us when it is deficient in calcium. It tells us by giving us cramping of the leg muscles or muscle spasms of the toes and feet, which inevitably affect sleep. Difficulty in falling asleep or not being able to sleep through the night may be associated with a calcium deficiency. Another cruel symptom of calcium deficiency is menstrual cramping. Most all of these symptoms can be corrected by augmenting the diet with foods that are high in calcium. Otherwise, a calcium supplement is necessary.

71

CHEWING

How could something like chewing change an entire family's life? When I entered my store one afternoon I was greeted by my coworker, who was helping a customer. It was her "Hello, Bob" that prompted the customer to ask if I was Bob Cannon. Smiling, my employee answered yes.

The customer, who introduced herself as Ruth, asked if she could shake my hand. I extended mine, expecting a formal handshake. Instead, she took my hand and held it in both of hers. Her eyes filled with tears as she thanked me for, as she said, "Changing the lives of my entire family."

Ruth said it had happened a year before. She had asked her daughter Pam to pick up some vitamins.

Pam came into my store with her four-year-old son, Mikey. While Pam was shopping, her son found the toy bin we had for the children. I noticed that Mikey was chewing the toys made out of wood. I asked his mother if he was teething. Without elaborating, Pam answered no.

I could have accepted Pam's answer and continued helping with her purchase, but it wasn't my style to accept a simple answer. Instead I asked questions to see the whole picture. After I had asked several questions about Mikey, Pam told me the whole the story.

He was always chewing on wood. Sometimes he would chew on a toy, a chair, the headboard of his crib, a table, or even a wooden spoon. If an object was made of wood, he would chew on it. She and her husband were so worried that they took him to the pediatrician. The doctor put Mikey on some medication to calm his nerves. After a couple of weeks, it was determined that the medication didn't work except to make Mikey sleep a lot. In fact, he slept too much. They returned to the doctor's office and told him. The doctor then intimated that there was a problem with Mikey's home life, specifically with his parents, and suggested they see a counselor. Pam and her husband decided to fire the doctor and seek a specialist for their son.

The specialist prescribed a different type of medication. That didn't work either; but now, instead of a sleepy little boy, Mikey became withdrawn and isolated. The doctor concluded that Mikey would eventually outgrow the problem and recommended that the parents take their son to a pediatric dentist friend so Mikey could be fitted for braces. In this way, Mikey would not ruin his teeth or, possibly, injure himself

They fired the specialist, too.

In desperation, they went to an internationally known medical center in our area for help. After several appointments, the team of doctors concluded that Mikey should be given therapy. This four-year-old boy was to see a psychologist.

I asked Pam if she would consider something in addition to the proposed therapy. She answered yes. It was time to ask more questions directly from my Body Language Questionnaire. I asked her about Mikey's diet. What did he eat, when did he eat, what were his favorite foods and his sleep routine?

Her answers led me to the conclusion that Mikey probably chewed on wood because he was deficient in minerals. I suggested that Pam buy some minerals and add them to his diet. She chose a multiple mineral formula in capsule form. Pam could open the capsule and add the contents to his juice. She bought the item, thanked me for the suggestion, and left the store.

Ruth told me the rest of the story. "As soon as my daughter got to my home, she told me what you had said and showed me the bottle of minerals. I told her that it seemed logical, but my daughter decided to confer with the doctors first to make sure it was indeed safe to give Mikey the minerals. The doctors said that it was too high a potency for a four-year-old and advised against the theory and the minerals. They added that Pam was wasting her money and that she shouldn't listen to charlatans when it came to the health of her child."

Ruth finally took one of her hands from mine and wiped the tears from her cheeks. Then she apologized for repeating how the doctors had referred to me.

I smiled and said that it was okay.

She continued her story. "That evening, Pam and I discussed with our husbands what the doctors had told us. We decided to go with your suggestion, but to give Mikey just half of the capsule. For the first time in almost a year, he slept soundly the whole night. And he wasn't sleepy throughout the next day. For that reason alone—a full night's sleep—we decided to give him a whole capsule. The next day at dinnertime we emptied it into some milk. Again he slept all night. Pam had to go home, but she promised to give Mikey another mineral capsule that evening. She called me the next day and reported that Mikey had slept all night and hadn't chewed on any wood since the previous afternoon.

"Pam asked me, 'Could this be the answer to his chewing? Is it possible that, after seeing all of these doctors, Mikey's problem was just the lack of minerals my vitamin guy suggested?'"

Still holding on to my hand, tears streaming down her cheeks, Ruth said that Mikey was all better.

He never chewed on wood again, he never needed medication, and he certainly didn't need therapy.

She thanked me once again.

I responded, "You're welcome. Oh, by the way, are your hands always so cold?"

72

Sweating and Energy

I have been told countless times that women don't sweat. In fact, they don't even perspire. They glisten with moisture.

There are always exceptions to the rule, and Donna was that exception. She was covered with sweat from her head down to the bottom of her—appropriately called—sweats.

She explained that she had just finished an extensive workout at the gym with her new trainer. "No pain, no gain, and I'm beginning to feel the pain already. In fact, I'm beginning to drag, and I have a twelve-hour work shift ahead of me."

Donna was a registered nurse who, at middle age, was determined to get into and stay in shape. "No middle-age spread for me," she repeated this motto between groans. "No pain, no gain, and no middle-age spread for me." She looked at me with tired eyes. "Oh gosh, Bob, I don't know if I can take it. Maybe it would be easier if I had a husband, no, better yet, a boyfriend. That would give me the incentive I need." We laughed together at her statement.

Donna had been a customer of mine even before her divorce. Together, we made her life more livable in spite of the trauma of the dissolution of a twelve-year marriage. Based on my advice, she took minerals to help her sleep, the amino acid L-phenylalanine to lessen her anguish, and the additional B-complex vitamins to help her with the stress. She made it through the divorce a stronger and healthier person. I complimented her when she told me that she was about to undertake training at the gym. I did not, however, agree with the philosophy of "No pain, no gain."

After completing her purchase, Donna lingered, while I waited on several other customers. She was obviously tired, perhaps even exhausted. I asked her if she was okay.

"I'm beat. I feel like I spent all my energy at the gym. But I've got to go to work, so I'll see you next week, Bob. Say hi to your wife for me." She got up and started for the door.

"Hold on, Donna, I was just taking a break. Would you care to join me? The drinks are on me."

"Thank you. I could use a drink. I have worked up a thirst."

I went to the back room and returned with two cups in my hands and handed one to Donna.

"What's this foamy stuff? It smells good." She took a sip and added, "It tastes good, but the fizzle got in my nose," she said as she tweaked her nose with her fingers. When another customer entered the store, I excused myself while Donna slowly sipped her drink. After several minutes, she said goodbye.

I watched her slowly get into her car. She sat there without starting the engine. After several minutes, she got out of the car and came back into my store asking, "Hey! What was in that drink you gave me?"

"Why?"

"I'm actually feeling better. I'm getting my energy back."

I smiled at her and walked toward a display of Emergen-C and showed her a packet.

"It's just vitamin C in powder form."

"It must be more than vitamin C. What does it contain to make it taste so good and give me my energy back?"

"It's loaded with the electrolyte minerals, especially potassium."

"Bob, I am a nurse and I did not recognize this potassium deficiency. You're good."

"I suspected a potassium deficiency based on your profuse sweating, your weakness or lack of energy, and your thirst. It was an educated guess. But even if I had been wrong, the drink would not harm you in any way."

73

SWALLOWING

He was a long-distance runner who competed regularly. He was in his fifties, had a slight build, and looked to be in fine condition. This day I noticed he was swallowing constantly, which prompted me to ask some questions.

"Do you have a sore throat or is your mouth just too dry?"

"Oh, my mouth feels like cotton. I've had this condition since my last race in Vegas."

"Did you ask your coach about it?" I knew the coach of his team was both a long-distance runner and a medical doctor.

"He told me to drink more water."

"Have you been checked for any specific conditions such as diabetes, salivary gland infection, or are you on any prescription drugs?"

"Yeah, he ran a series of tests before the last two major races. I'm okay, just a dry mouth."

"How about leg cramps," I asked.

"Yes, I have been getting leg cramps lately, so I increased my minerals, especially calcium, but it hasn't helped much."

"How about feelings of weakness or tiredness?"

Again I got an affirmative answer.

"Have you been craving any particular foods lately, specifically bananas, baked potatoes, or dried fruit?"

"Bananas. How did you know that? I seem to be craving them; in fact, I probably eat three or four a day."

"Does your dry mouth lessen after eating that many bananas?"

He answered no and added that he was feeling rather weak and should go home.

"If you're that weak, how about a drink of water?"

"That's okay, I have some in the car."

"It's probably hot water by now. I'll get you some. Do you mind if I put Emergen-C in it?"

He answered that it would be fine, in fact, he added, he had heard about it but had never tried it. I offered him the glass of water with the bubbling Emergen-C.

First he sipped it, said that it tasted pretty good, and then chug-a-lugged the remaining liquid. I thought it was best for him to stay awhile, rather than go outside in the extreme heat.

After talking for a few minutes, he asked if he could have another glass of Emergen-C. He drank the second glass slowly, almost as if he was savoring its contents. After a short while he asked, "Why did you offer me this Emergen-C?"

Answer a question with a question, I was once taught. "What do you mean?"

"I'm feeling better. In fact, I don't have that weak feeling anymore. Could it have been the Emergen-C? I'm feeling much better. Maybe I should buy a box. It really tastes good."

"Why don't you ask your doctor/coach if you should take some potassium; you might be low. You certainly have the signs of a deficiency, and Emergen-C has potassium plus the electrolytes."

"That's why I was craving the bananas!" he exclaimed. "And you knew it, that's why you offered me the Emergen-C. That is the reason, isn't it?"

"Naw. You just looked thirsty," I teased. "Anyway, if I had offered you the Emergen-C for your feelings of weakness it could have been construed that I was prescribing and, since I'm not a physician, I certainly can't prescribe." I added, however, that it was probably a good idea to buy the box of Emergen-C, and he did. A few weeks later he was pleased to tell me that he found additional information about his condition on the Internet. He was positive that he had a potassium deficiency due to the amount of sweating he did, especially in the last race in the desert community of Las Vegas.

"We're always told to take salt tablets, but never potassium. From now on I'm going to include Emergen-C in my running kit."

All this took place because I observed his need to continually swallow. His body was crying out for potassium.

74

ATTENTION DEFICIT DISORDER (ADD)

"Look. Look what you've done to my son!"

Everyone in the store heard her loud voice, including my employees and my customers. Her manner convinced me that she wanted everyone to hear her, and everyone did stop to listen to her and what she was about to say.

"I came in here last week just to buy some vitamins, and you, you Bob, suggested that I buy, no, you gave me the pills, and I gave them to my little David. I trusted you and look what happened to him. In less than a week, my little boy has become tolerable. Tolerable. How can I ever thank you?" she asked.

The tears that had been streaming down her face changed to heavy sobbing. One of my employees walked over and placed her arm around Miriam's shoulders and just held her until her crying lessened.

Through her tears she said to her son, "David, go thank Mr. Bob for helping you get better."

David, who had just turned six, walked toward me, extending his hand to mine. His hand was still just as moist as I remembered from last week. I asked little David to give me a high five to confirm my suspicions.

Miriam, David, and David's little sister, Rachel, had indeed been in my store last week—Miriam, to buy some vitamins; Rachel, to play with the toys I have to keep little children occupied; and David was there to destroy the store! He took the toys from Rachel and threw them down the aisles. He removed, no, he yanked vitamin bottles off the shelves and pushed them into other shelves, creating a mess. He tried stacking five- and ten-pound containers of protein powder, only to push them over and yell, "Timber!" David had been a menace. That was when my employee called me up front to help with David. I was to keep watch over him so that his mother could shop.

While playing the role of babysitter, I asked Miriam a myriad of questions about David.

"Bob, he has been diagnosed with so many problems—ADD, ADHD, plus several other conditions. If he were in his fifties, with all of the letters after his name, he would appear to be a well-educated person. Instead, he has all of these afflictions."

I knew David was adopted; thus, Miriam had no history of his parents and what illnesses they might have had. She and the many doctors David was seeing were perplexed about why David wasn't responding to the many medications that were usually prescribed for these conditions. I asked David to give me a high five. I had to find out if the palms of his hands were moist. My suspicions were correct—his hand was moist, very moist.

"Miriam, since you don't have a family history of your son, couldn't we presume that he was put up for adoption because his parents, or parent, was either an alcoholic, on drugs, or both?" Because of his moist hands, I assumed he had inherited a blood sugar problem from one or both of his parents.

"Bob, that's what my husband and I suspected. Hopefully, his parents decided that David needed a better home than they could provide. Unfortunately, we haven't been able to provide that for him. Oh, he gets our love and attention, but we cannot control his temperament. And he's doing so poorly in school. David is not dumb; in fact, he's very smart. His problem is not being able to sit still. That's when the teacher diagnosed Attention Deficit Disorder (ADD). Bob, I say that sarcastically. I know teachers can't diagnose, it's illegal, but I believe they influence the doctor's diagnosis with their opinion. Anyway, the doctor then confirmed it."

"Unfortunately, Miriam, we hear of so many instances where the teacher suggested to the parents that their child might have this condition."

"Then it's not just my opinion?"

Instead of answering, I asked another question. "What's his diet like? What does he eat?"

"He won't eat anything except cookies, candy, and soda pop. He refuses to eat his vegetables, spits out meat, any kind of meat, and knocks his glass of milk over if we try to get him to drink it. He has become an unbearable child, but we won't give up. We won't give him back. Someone has to help him; unfortunately, says my husband, "It has to be us."

"What is his sleep pattern and what is his temperament?"

"David refuses to go to sleep. He stays awake until eleven or sometimes twelve o'clock. His temperament? He screams, yells, and throws temper tantrums. Then he cries and says he's sorry. Bob, you suggested that his parents might have been alcoholic or maybe even drug addicts. Is there a reason you reached that conclusion, or is it just speculation?"

"Miriam, when I asked David to give me a high five, it was to determine if his hand was moist."

"Oh, they're always wet. You could have asked me that. Bob, is there any parallel between moist hands and alcohol or drugs?"

I told her there was. Before she could ask what could be done, I suggested she complete the Body Language Questionnaire for David.

"I will. I promise. But what will it tell me?"

We discussed the possibility of David's being deficient in minerals, pantothenic acid, and the B vitamins and the role they play in behavioral problems.

"I wish I could buy them all, and right now, but my husband doesn't believe in vitamins like I do. Somehow I'll have to convince him that supplements can help our son. I won't be able to buy anything until he agrees."

I walked over to the sport section of my store and removed a bottle from the shelf.

"Here, take this with my compliments. In that way, you can honestly tell your husband that you didn't buy it. It's L-glutamine. It's an amino acid, similar to the L-lysine that you took for your cold sore problem, only L-glutamine has other benefits."

"Are you going to tell me these benefits, or do I have to ask?"

"Some people use it to lessen their cravings for sugar, which includes alcohol, of course. Others use it as a brain food. Some use it to enable them to focus their brain or their thoughts. David, because of his age, would take less than one-fourth of the dosage recommended for adults."

Miriam accepted my gift for David, and together the three of them left the store. My employees and I spent the next half-hour straightening out the mess David had created. When Miriam returned the following week along with David, my employees and I were not very eager to see him, even though he was just a little boy. When Miriam said, "Look what you've done to my son," I could see joy in her eyes, even through the tears. She continued with her story.

"Bob, after you gave me the L-glutamine pills last week, I showed them to my husband. Initially he said no, but, after seeing the hope in my eyes, he reluctantly agreed to give them to David for one week and one week only. That was Thursday. The following Tuesday, as we were retiring for the night, my husband said that he had observed significant changes in David. The next day, David's teacher called, commenting that the medication for David was finally working. 'He's more attentive in class and he just earned an A in reading.' Reading is David's least favorite subject in school, and he just got an A! I couldn't wait for my husband to get home, so I called him at work and told him what the teacher had shared with me. He cried, Bob, he cried just like a baby. I have never heard or seen my husband cry. We both knew it was the L-glutamine and not the drugs. My husband agrees that I should buy whatever this Questionnaire determines our son to be deficient in."

One year later, after dramatic dietary changes and supplementation, David was no longer taking medication for his illnesses. He became a straight-A student and was promoted an additional grade the next semester. His doctors? When Miriam told them what she had been doing this past year—the change in his diet, giving him vitamin and mineral supplements, and her taking David off the medication—the doctors collectively agreed that David's illnesses, all of them, were undoubtedly misdiagnosed.

75

I CAN TALK NOW

Our children learned about nutrition from my wife and me, of course, and it was my younger daughter who suggested L-glutamine to her friend Karen. Karen's four-year-old son, Johnny, could say words, but he had difficulty forming sentences. He would say a word, pause for a moment, say a second word, pause for another moment, and then continue to the next word, always pausing between words. The best he could do, sentence-wise, was "goodnight" or "bye, bye." Even "I love you, Mommy" was too difficult for him to say without pausing. The other children in Johnny's class were starting to make fun of the way he talked. For awhile Johnny laughed with them, but lately he tried to ask, in his deliberate way, "Why are they always laughing at me?"

Through the doctor, Karen had tried various kinds of medication. At first they thought it could be stress, but that was quickly ruled out. Then they tried a speech therapist, but to no avail. The therapist identified Johnny as a slow learner who might or might not grow out of it, and said it would take years to find out. That's when my daughter Cathy suggested L-glutamine.

"Karen," she said, "empty the contents of one capsule into some juice and divide this into four doses. One in the morning before breakfast, the second one at bedtime, the third and fourth for the next day, and always on an empty stomach. And don't give it to him with milk—only juice or water."

At first Karen was a little reluctant to give such a high potency to her four-year-old son, but eventually she decided to try the L-glutamine. The information Cathy had given her about the amino acid convinced Karen that it was safe, even for her young son.

Less than a week later, Karen called Cathy saying that someone wanted to talk to her. That's when she put Johnny on the telephone. He said, "Hi, Auntie Cathy. How are you? Mommy and I are having fun. We are reading a lot of books. Bye, Auntie Cathy. I love you."

When Karen got back on the telephone she was crying and so was Cathy. She told my daughter that when she put little Johnny to bed the night before, he looked up at her and said, without any hesitation, "Goodnight, Mommy. Mommy, I love you and Daddy so much."

L-glutamine, like most amino acids, should be taken on an empty stomach, or, at the least, on a protein-empty stomach. Furthermore, vitamins B-6 and C enhance the absorption of most amino acids.

76

I Can't Read

"C,c,can--you--you--find--Wil--Wil--Willie? He--He--He's--un..."

With apparent disgust, she put down the book and reached for a game instead.

I had at my store a box that included toys, games, puzzles, and books to keep children occupied while their parents shopped. This little girl, Lindsey, was twelve years old and could barely read. I overheard her trying to read the story of Willie, but it was with extreme difficulty so she gave up and put the book down. When her mother approached the checkout counter, Lindsey joined her. Upon the completion of the sale, the mother began writing out her check. That's when I asked Lindsey to spell the word *vitamin.*

The little girl said, "I can't read, and I don't know how to spell."

The mother looked up at me and asked, "Are you trying to embarrass my daughter?"

Instead of answering her question, I began telling a short story. "A few years ago, a customer was writing her check, just as you are doing, when she hesitated on writing the word *vitamin.* I spelled the word for her and told her that I have three schoolteachers who also have difficulty spelling that word. The customer stopped writing, looked up at me, and said, 'Four.' Yes, she too was a schoolteacher. My point is that the word *vitamin* is difficult to spell. Perhaps it's difficult because of the many ways that it is abbreviated: *vit*, *vite*, or *vita*."

"What does that have to do with my daughter?"

"I noticed that she was having a difficult time reading one of my storybooks. Perhaps I can help." I did not wait for approval to ask a series of questions. Does she have a specific eye problem? Does she require glasses? Does she have dyslexia? Instead of answering each question, the mother told me that Lindsey just had great difficulty in reading and writing. She was above average in the rest of her classes.

I told them a story about my own mother and that of little Johnny, the son of my daughter's best friend, and a product called L-glutamine. Then I asked the mother if she would be willing to consider buying what I had suggested.

"What did you call that product, again?" she asked.

"L-glutamine. It's an amino acid, which is considered 'brain fuel.'"

"What is an amino acid?"

"You are familiar with the alphabet, of course. And that it has twenty-six letters. The twenty-six letters make up the alphabet. Protein is made up of twenty-eight amino acids. Together, these appriximately twenty-eight amino acids make up protein. L-glutamine is just one of the amino acids that make up protein as, say, the letter *a* is one of the letters of the alphabet."

"And L-glutamine will help Lindsey to read?"

"Based on previous experiences, yes, it could. There are always exceptions, of course, but if Lindsey's problem is what they call a 'lazy brain,' then she will be helped. Again, based on previous experiences, results can be determined within the week."

This was Monday. On Friday afternoon I heard the results of the L-glutamine. Lindsey had received a B+ on her most recent spelling exam. She usually received D's and F's.

The mother asked, "Can we expect these results from now on?"

"Yes," I answered, and by the end of the school year, L-glutamine proved me right.

77

MEMORY

If only I had known about the amino acid L-glutamine when I was attending school, perhaps my grades would have been better. Now when I talk to someone who is about to take a test, I suggest that he or she consider L-glutamine.

I proposed this amino acid to a student attending California State University at Davis. Studying to become a veterinarian, she was a typical stressed-out student. I sold her the L-glutamine because her diet was insufficient in many ways. I also sold her a liquid protein called Cheramino. This liquid protein contains all of the essential amino acids that might have been lacking in her diet. An inadequate supply of even one essential amino acid can hinder the synthesis and reduce body levels of necessary proteins.

It worked! Not only did her grades improve significantly, but so did her physical and mental energy levels. Yes, she did graduate and is now practicing in California's San Fernando Valley.

Another customer was studying to become a beautician. Although she was doing well in most of her studies, there were two areas where she was failing. Because of poor diet, she too took both the L-glutamine and the Cheramino. On the day following her finals, she called to tell me her test results.

"Bob," she said, "my plan was to do the difficult part for the first two hours and the easier part in the last hour. But then, the answers just came to me, especially those I thought would be the most difficult. I couldn't believe what was happening. I finished the entire test in less than two hours! Yes, I passed. It was a breeze!"

78

ALZHEIMER'S

At age seventy-five, Mom was living in a nursing home and was mostly confined to her bed. After experiencing many mini-strokes, she suffered from both dementia and Alzheimer's, according to her doctors. On occasions, and these were becoming more rare, she would recognize her family and was able to communicate with us as long as we talked about things that happened many years ago. It was terribly frustrating to see this once-vibrant woman mentally deteriorating before our eyes. Could L-glutamine help?

I had read many articles written by renowned authors about this amino acid. Many studies concluded that supplemental L-glutamine could be helpful in treating senility and developmental problems, and because it can pass the blood-brain barrier, it is considered a brain fuel. Would it help my mother? I discussed its merits with my stepfather, hoping to convince him to try it with Mom. He said no. I didn't pursue it any further with him, as we didn't agree on most things anyway. But I could pursue it on my own without telling him or my brother and sister. I decided that I would initiate my plan the next day, Sunday.

Upon arriving at the nursing home, I checked to see if my stepfather or any of my siblings were present before I entered Mom's room. Good, she was by herself, lying there in a fetal position. I called to her and, surprisingly, she somewhat responded, although she didn't recognize me. I helped her into a sitting position, and, after mixing the equivalent of ten L-glutamine capsules into water, I brought the glass to her mouth for her to drink. And she did!

Ten capsules of L-glutamine totaled 5,000 mg. According to the experts, this was considered an overdose if consumed over a prolonged period of time. I knew that it wouldn't be, of course, and I needed a dose large enough to get a result. Hopefully, a positive one. On Monday, the next day, I repeated the procedure using the same amount of L-glutamine.

While on my lunch hour Tuesday, I visited my mom again. As I entered her room I first saw my sister, who greeted me warmly. My stepfather was sitting next to Mom's bed. It was empty! My mind started to race, but my thoughts were interrupted by my mother asking, "Bobby, my baby. Is that you?"

She was sitting in a wheelchair, and because of her recent loss of eyesight, couldn't readily see me. "Bobby, my baby. Is that you?" Her words reverberated in my mind. I couldn't hold back the tears as I walked over to her for a hug. This was a miracle happening before my eyes! Mom recognized me!

I looked at my sister, who was also crying, and then at my stepfather, and while still holding my mother, said to him, "See, Pop, I told you vitamins could help!" Although I said "vitamins" to him, I really meant improved nutrition, and, of course, L-glutamine. The lunch hour I spent with my mother and sister was glorious.

My stepfather? He still maintained his negative attitude about nutrition and life in general.

On Wednesday's lunch hour, I was ready to resume the L-glutamine therapy, as I wasn't able to give Mom any while my stepfather was present.

"Mr. Weiss." Someone with a very stern voice called my name.

"Yes?"

"Mr. Weiss, I have specific instructions from Mr. Rose (my stepfather) and the doctor, restraining you from giving any vitamins to his wife."

She emphasized "his wife," rather than saying "your mother." My stepfather was undoubtedly in charge of my mother's well-being.

Would my mother have continuously improved from the L-glutamine? I never did find out, as the restrictions placed by my stepfather continued through her death.

79

Cold Sores

When I was a pre-teenager and teenager, I suffered—I mean *really* suffered—from cold sores. Not only were they an annoyance, but they also hurt, and, most of all, they were embarrassing. The more embarrassed I got, the more cold sores I got. Sometimes they would cover both my upper and lower lips. It was vicious. How many times was the question raised while I was in class at school, "Teacher, what is that odor?" Yes, it was from me. I tried to apply my campho-something or other without being too conspicuous, but the odor always gave me away.

"Robert's got pimples on his lips," they would say laughingly.

Why did they always call me Robert when the rest of the time they called me Bob? Anyway, they weren't pimples, they were cold sores. Unfortunately I didn't learn about L-lysine, an amino acid, until I got in the health food industry at the age of forty. I endured almost thirty years of hurting until I read about L-lysine. No, it wasn't every day that I got cold sores, and sometimes they wouldn't appear for months, but when they did it was with a vengeance, and it seemed an eternity before they would finally disappear.

Several years ago I met with my sister and brother at a restaurant to discuss family matters. As we settled into our seats, our waitress came over to take our order. I looked at her lips, specifically her lower lip. It had two ugly sores on it, clearly visible in spite of the dimmed lighting.

She took our drink orders: coffee for my sister, and my brother and I had cranberry juice.

"Bladder infections?" she asked jokingly.

I'm sure she was sorry she made the quip, as it made us all laugh, including her. Then she grimaced with pain caused by the sores on her lip. She had tried covering her lower lip with her upper lip when she asked for our order, but when we laughed she revealed that awful scourge, cold sores! She confirmed our order and quickly turned away, perhaps to keep us from seeing her affliction, and started toward her station.

"Well, she seems to know about vitamins; at least she knows that cranberry juice is good for bladder infections," my sister said.

Apparently my sister and brother had not seen her affliction, as neither of them commented on it. We were in the middle of our family discussion when the waitress returned with our drinks. She was still trying to cover up the sore on her lower lip using her upper lip—something that those of us who suffered with cold sores know how to do. I wondered if she, too, had suffered with cold sores all through school the way I had. I would guess that she might have suffered even more, because she was very attractive and probably popular in school. More people meant more exposure, which may have caused her more embarrassment.

Should I tell her about L-lysine? Should I make her aware that her problem is correctable? How would she react? Would she be upset, embarrassed, perhaps even angry?

My brother brought me back to the family discussion by asking my opinion about something. It was the second time he had asked the question, since I hadn't heard him the first time. My thoughts were on the waitress and her dilemma, and I was reliving some of my own pain and suffering from my school days.

After an hour or so we finished our family discussion, divided up the check, left the appropriate tip, and walked to the cashier's station.

"I'll be right back," I said to my family.

"What's the matter?" my brother asked.

"I'll meet you outside." I hurried back to our table and wrote on the back of a napkin: *For cold sores. Take L-lysine, an amino acid, in 500 mg tablets. They can be purchased at any vitamin store.*

I couldn't leave without making her aware of L-lysine. I wasn't prescribing, just sharing information with another person who suffered from the same affliction. I took the napkin and wrapped it around the tip we had left for her. As I was putting it down, I noticed that she was heading in my direction, so I turned and once again headed toward the exit. Just outside the door I heard her call to me.

"Sir. Mister, please wait."

My brother and sister heard her, too, and turned around to see what was going on.

"Mister. I mean sir." She had finally caught up with me, and, holding the napkin in her hand, she pointed toward what I had written.

The waitress asked me, "Is it true? Will this stuff help with my cold sores? My doctor said it was incurable. Are you a doctor?"

"No, I'm not a doctor, but I suffered from cold sores throughout junior and senior high school. I know the hurt."

"Were you laughed at and ridiculed too?" she asked.

"Yes, I was, and I also know how much they can hurt, especially when you laugh or smile. No, I'm not a doctor, but it was a doctor, actually a dentist, who made me aware of this therapy. As for incurable, perhaps it is, but L-lysine will, at the very least, arrest it and keep you from suffering."

Both anguish and joy were in her voice as she said, "I've suffered with these sores my entire life, especially in school and when dating." Then she asked the hard question: "Does this L-lysine really work? Am I getting my hopes up prematurely? What else can I do to keep them from happening?"

She really wanted answers. I looked at my sister and brother; they both were interested in helping the waitress. In the light I could see that her nametag said Monica.

"Monica, I used to get cold sores four or five times a year, sometimes even more. Now, if I feel one coming on, and you know what I mean, I start taking L-lysine throughout the day and always an hour before eating. Watch your intake of nuts and chocolate. Avoid excess stress and excess exposure to sunlight. Yes, your problem will end."

"Sir, there have been times when I received a hundred-dollar tip just for bringing someone a drink. As nice and as needed as the money was, this is the best tip I have ever received. Thank you."

The look in her eyes and in the eyes of countless others when they learn that there is help for their conditions makes the embarrassment of telling strangers how to correct their problems worthwhile.

80

L-LYSINE OR B-2?

Several weeks before, a young man who had been looking in the sports section of my store said he was trying to find L-lysine. I noticed the sores in the corners of his mouth.

"Why the L-lysine?" I asked.

He said he was going to try it one more time even though it hadn't really helped him in the past.

"Hadn't helped with what?" I asked, since he had not really answered my first question.

"Oh, my doctor said I should use L-lysine for my cold sores, but it didn't really do that much in healing them. They usually go away in two or three months on their own, but I thought that maybe, maybe, I wasn't taking enough of them. How many do you suggest I take, and when?"

"Probably not any at all," I answered.

He looked up from the bottle in his hand and asked, "You mean L-lysine doesn't work for this? I was surprised when my doctor suggested it, especially when he told me to go to a vitamin store. I thought it was a prescription drug. Maybe I shouldn't buy this after all." With that he put the bottle back on the shelf.

"Are you prone to cold sores?" I asked. When he answered yes, I asked him where on his lips they usually were located.

He answered that they were always in the corners of his mouth.

"I noticed your eyes are red. Do you work on the computer a lot or do you wear contacts?"

"Yes to all three. Why?"

First, I told him he was fortunate to have a medical doctor recommending something other than a prescription drug. Unfortunately, however, the diagnosis might not have been correct. I asked him the usual questions relevant to a B-2 deficiency—red eyes, burning and/or itching eyes, and depression.

He answered yes to all but the question about depression. He said his only depression was that these sores didn't clear up.

I told him that his answers indicated he probably had a vitamin B-2 deficiency, and sores in the corner of the mouth were just another indication of the same deficiency.

"B-2? But I take a B-12 complex, isn't that enough of the B's?"

"What is a B-12 complex?" I asked myself. It's either B-12 singularly or all of the vitamins. The latter is referred to as a B-complex, which includes B-12.

"Apparently the potency of your vitamin is low; otherwise, this B-2 deficiency wouldn't occur."

"Okay, you're the boss; you certainly seem to know what you are talking about. I'll try anything to get rid of these things, but will I have to take B-2 for the rest of my life?"

"Probably not. In fact, once you correct the problem, your multiple vitamin should act as a maintenance dose. Bring your B-12 complex to me so I can evaluate it."

He bought the B-2, but wouldn't consider an additional B-complex. He called two weeks later telling me that his mouth problem was gone, but he still was concerned that it would come back again.

I reminded him again to bring in his B-12 complex so I could evaluate it; perhaps it wasn't adequate for his lifestyle.

He said he would, but I never saw him again. His B-12 complex was probably just vitamin B-12; otherwise, the B-2 deficiency would not have occurred. Hopefully, someday someone will convince him that he needs to take an additional B-complex or a multiple vitamin when taking B vitamins individually.

81

SKIN - SENSITIVITY TO THE SUN

"Hiding in your tent is not a fun vacation," I told this first-time customer who had come into my store with her friend, Alana, a regular customer. They were discussing their upcoming vacation at the Colorado River that would include fishing, swimming, boating, and water skiing. Alana's friend said she wasn't able to do any of the fun things, because she was both blonde and fair-skinned, which made her extremely sensitive to the sun. This is how the conversation began.

I asked Alana what I could help her find. She answered that she knew where everything was but that I should help her friend. The blonde-haired woman was a nurse who absolutely didn't believe in my industry and told me so.

"Don't bother me with this nonsense. Alana is crazy if she thinks that these pills can help her in any way. They're just a bunch of placebos."

Ouch! I thought it would be nice if she and other unbelievers could spend a day in my store and see the positive results supplements achieve in advancing health. But she had declared war with me, so I decided to go on the offensive. "Too bad you won't be able to enjoy the sun with the rest of your friends," I said.

I assumed that, because she was fair-skinned, she wouldn't be able to cope with the blazing hot Colorado sun.

"While they burn their bodies, I will find the best shade possible and catch up with my reading."

"Hiding in your tent is not a fun vacation. What if you could get out in the sun without it burning your skin? Wouldn't you prefer that to reading?"

"Sunblock doesn't work for me. I still burn. I will be pale-white forever. At least I have an all-over white tan, no strap marks or such."

"Let's see. You burn easily, you're sensitive to the sun, and I noticed a little white blotch on your upper arm."

"That?" she said, pointing to an area about the size of a quarter. "That's something that just happened about two years ago. The doctor said it's not malignant; it's just, as you called it, a blotch on the skin. It's not getting any worse, or better for that matter. I hope you're not going to tell me it's a deficiency of a vitamin or something. I'm not that gullible."

I didn't answer her but instead turned and walked toward the vitamin B section of the store, picked up a bottle, and returned to where she was standing.

"Here. Prove me right or prove me wrong." It was a challenge that I hoped she would accept. I put the bottle in her hand.

"What's PABA?"

"It's a B vitamin that I believe will prove me right. Take it, try it, and when it works, that's when you come back and pay me. Most people in your situation take one pill with each meal, for the duration of their vacation. So take it, and venture out in the sun. Be reasonable, though. Only stay out for an hour or less. You'll know if it's working."

I took the bottle from her, put it in a bag, and handed it back to her. I then turned to Alana, my regular customer, who, after hearing my challenge to her friend the nurse, was smiling. She didn't make any comment about the PABA but winked and showed me her crossed fingers, obviously hoping that the PABA would work.

The nurse did return after her vacation, first to pay me and, second, to show off her first-time suntan! She, too, had become a believer in vitamins and was to be a regular customer for several years. After doing extensive research on her own, she discovered that the little blotch on her skin, as well as her premature graying, could be associated with a deficiency of PABA.

82

Swimmer's Ear

One afternoon a father came into the store with his daughter. While he was being helped by one of my co-workers I noticed that his daughter, who was in her very early teens, just stood quietly near the front door. I also noticed that she kept putting her hand up to her ear, but without touching it. Her eyes were very red. The combination of red eyes and her apparent ear sensitivity prompted me to ask, "Swimmer's ear?"

"Yes," she answered.

"Do you get it frequently?"

"Yes, I'm on a swim team, well maybe not for long if this ear thing keeps happening."

"Don't you wear ear plugs? If they are a good fit they usually help prevent it."

"They don't always help. I guess it's because I spend so much time under water. I mean, on the swim team it seems as if we're under water more than we are above it. Maybe it's the water pressure that causes them to leak."

"What do you know about swimmer's ear?" asked her father, who had overheard our conversation.

"I know it can be very painful and that you must be careful not to get an infection in the middle-ear, which is a lot more serious. Otherwise it is a rather benign situation. Is she on any antibiotics?" I asked.

"Not this time, at least not yet," replied the father.

"I had a conversation this morning with a mother about her daughter and gave her some suggestions for her daughter's problem."

"I'm interested. Anything that can be done to even lessen the problem would be helpful. We're hoping they don't drop her from the swim team."

"This is what my customer bought for her daughter this morning," I said as I handed him a bottle of vitamin A, a bottle of Sovereign Silver, and a package of ear candles.

I explained the importance of vitamin A in preventing infections in any of the body's orifices, including the ear. The Sovereign Silver brand of colloidal silver has a reputation for correcting almost any kind of minor infection, and the ear candles draw the water from the ear canal. He was somewhat astonished, especially about the ear candles.

"Wow, won't your mother be shocked when I tell her that we have finally found a solution to your problem? How can I ever thank you?" he asked.

He bought the three items plus his regular purchase, and he and his daughter left the store.

Less than an hour later, I was called to the telephone. "Bob," said the caller. "I was in earlier and bought some things for my daughter's ear problem."

"Yes, of course

Have you had a chance to apply them?"

"No. She just got home. Her father picked her up at school and apparently went to your store. That's why I'm calling. My husband told me about this miracle solution that will correct our daughter's problem. He said that he bought it at your store and that a woman had been in earlier and bought the same things! Bob, that woman was me, and I can't break my husband's bubble! Can I return the ear remedies I bought?"

Chuckling to myself I told her, "Yes, of course." However, the mother never did return her original purchase. She learned there were several other swim team girls who occasionally had the same problem. She passed on her new knowledge of vitamin A as a preventative of infection, colloidal silver as a remedy for infection, and ear candles as a method of drawing water out of the ear.

83

Swollen Glands

As Missy was shopping, I showed her six-year-old son, Derek, our toy bin. That's when I noticed his neck, more specifically his glands located in the neck. They were extremely swollen.

"Missy," I asked, "are your son's glands always so swollen?"

In her southern accent she replied, "Yes, sir. He's had them for almost six months. He's been on all kinds of antibiotics, seen several different doctors, but without success. The current doctor said it was a losing battle, so he scheduled Derek for surgery. Apparently, the glands are so full of poisons that it's best they be removed. I cried for two days when they told me that. I can't see surgery for such a little boy, but they are the doctors. I guess they know what they're doing."

"Are you joking? Was the doctor just teasing you? Do they really want to do surgery on him? Missy, I can't believe it," I was shocked.

If the doctors really had decided on surgery, was it because they had failed to correct Derek's problem, and, if so, what's the next best thing to do? Get the glands out of the picture by removing them. Cut them out. Get them out of the way.

"Missy, when is Derek scheduled for surgery?" I asked, still in disbelief.

"After the doctor gets back from vacation. That's four weeks from now."

"Would you consider something other than surgery? Something more natural?"

"Do you mean vitamins could help him? Isn't it too late? I mean, the doctor said that Derek's condition has become very serious."

"That's why he's doing the surgery after he enjoys his vacation?" There was a certain amount of contempt in my voice, and Missy heard it.

"That's what I thought too, Bob. If Derek's condition is so serious, why wait? Why not do the surgery tomorrow?"

"Because fate has stepped in. Maybe with the doctor going on vacation, it gave you a chance to correct Derek's condition yourself. Before the surgery. Let me show you what I have in mind." Together we walked over to several unopened boxes.

"These boxes contain an item called a re-bounder. It's actually a mini-trampoline. It's being promoted as a machine for losing weight by bouncing on it. In that way, people can get their exercise. This might help Derek with his swollen glands. At least, I believe it has merit."

"You mean bouncing on that thing will cure his problem?" There was a certain amount of skepticism in her voice, and rightly so.

"Missy, as you know, the heart pumps the blood to your body via the circulatory system. The lymphatic system, of which the glands are made, has no pump. The lymph system relies on the movement of the body, through walking, exercising, or flexing of the muscles to promote the passage of fluid. In Derek's case, the lymph system is clogged up and accumulating in his neck, causing his glands to swell. My theory is that by his bouncing on the mini-trampoline, he can clear out his glands and get his lymph system working again. Again, it's just a theory."

Was it doubt in her mind, or was she weighing what I had just told her?

"How much does the trampoline cost?" she asked.

"Look, Missy, I just got these in, and I'm supposed to have two of them as demos. Would you consider using one of my demos for a couple of weeks? In that way, it won't cost you anything, and it will prove or disprove my theory."

Missy accepted my proposition, so I loaded the mini-trampoline into her car. She called the next day telling me how much Derek enjoyed bouncing on it. Maybe it was the trampoline, maybe the antibiotics that finally overwhelmed the glandular infections. Whatever the reason, Derek improved dramatically over the next two weeks and was cleared of any infection within the month.

84

Eyes - Black or Bruised

I couldn't help but notice her black eye, even though she was trying to hide it behind huge sunglasses. The glasses were so dark that she was struggling to read the label on the herb bottle she was holding.

"Go ahead and take off your glasses. There's no one here but you and me, and I won't tell anyone."

Too forward, you say? If I see a situation or condition that I know is fixable through supplementation or whatever, I develop this boldness to say or ask. Rarely is the person offended. That was the case here.

"Oh, I'm so embarrassed about my eye. I thought I hid it rather well with these dark glasses. How did you see it? You must have X-ray vision or something."

"I'm just nosey, I guess. But it was the dark glasses, especially on an overcast day like this, that got me curious. I saw your eye as you were turning away from me. It's not that visible, really; I was just looking for some reason for the glasses."

"You are nosey, but I'm not offended." She took off her dark glasses, enabling me to see the full blunt of her eye. It was black, blue, and red, and it looked extremely painful.

"Dare I ask the cause?"

"Well, let's see. I walked into a door, I fell from an airplane, a horse kicked me, or my husband hit me." With the last statement, she looked to the floor.

"Anything broken? Have you been to the doctor?"

"Yes, the police took me to the emergency hospital after they arrested my husband."

All she wanted was some herbs. I could have gotten them for her, rung up her purchase, took her money, bagged the bottle, and said thank you and goodbye. Not me. I had to get nosier and ask more embarrassing questions. But if I hadn't, she wouldn't have learned about arnica montana, bioflavonoids, green tea, MSM, and Rescue Remedy, for which she gratefully thanked me.

Based on many customers' comments, these items, used separately or together, speed the healing process and limit pain.

Weeks later she explained about her husband. This was the only time in their marriage of fifteen years that he had ever struck her. For this reason, the judge placed him on probation. She added that he had had too much to drink and lost control. He'd been an angel since then and often asked her for forgiveness in spite of her repeated reassurances. She confided in me a couple of years later that her husband had become a born-again Christian and was truly angelic to both her and their children.

85

BAD BREATH - DOGS

One evening while my wife and I were taking a walk in our neighborhood, we met some neighbors who lived the next street over. While we were chatting with them, their collie came bounding out of the backyard. Of course, it sniffed at both my wife and me and then wanted to be petted. I obliged, especially around the ears and under the collar. That's when I noticed the dog's horrible breath. I could not help backing away.

The neighbors laughed. "Smells like spoiled eggs, doesn't she?" They laughed some more.

"Does she always have such bad breath or did you just feed her table scraps laced with garlic or something?"

"Naw, she always smells that way."

"She could have something seriously wrong with her. Have you considered taking her to a vet?"

"Yeah, we already did, but there's nothing wrong; she just has bad breath. The vet did give us some pills, but they didn't work. We're just going to have to live with it."

I suggested they try chlorophyll to make the dog more socially acceptable.

"If it works for the breath, as you say, do you know of anything that will keep the male dogs away while she's in heat?"

"I don't know of anything to keep the dogs away, but, according to the many dog breeders we have as customers, they use chlorophyll for that reason as well."

86

Eyes - Conjunctivitis

It was early one Saturday morning when a mother and her four children came into my store. They were first-time customers who came in because of a referral. The first thing I noticed was their behavior—it was admirable. Then I noticed the eyes of the youngest they were blood-red and oozing with pus. It was obvious that this child's condition was not caused by crying. As I approached the mother, I noticed that her eyes were also blood-red and oozing. It was very apparent that both mom and youngest child had a very bad eye infection. We exchanged greetings.

"A dear friend suggested I come to see you. You are Bob, aren't you?"

I answered yes and asked how I could help her.

"I, we, have been going to the doctor for over three months now, have spent well over four hundred dollars, and we still can't get rid of this eye infection. At the suggestion of our doctor we even vacated our home for a couple of weeks, thinking that something in the house might be the cause. Nothing has worked so far. I mentioned to my friend that I was going to try some eyebright herb. That's when she suggested that I go see Bob and talk to him or his staff because they're so knowledgeable. What do you think? I mean, what is your opinion about eyebright? I heard it works wonders."

"Oh my," I exclaimed.

"What's the matter?"

"I didn't notice the rest of the children's eyes. All of you have this same infection."

"Yes," she answered, "even my husband has it. He can't go to work, the children can't go to school, and I'm embarrassed to go to the market."

Three months and four hundred dollars and still no positive results. This eye condition, which she said the doctor diagnosed as conjunctivitis, is also associated with vitamin A and vitamin B-2 deficiencies. Unfortunately, it takes awhile for these vitamins to correct the problem. Eyebright is a wonderful herb. Besides taking it internally, most people use it as an eyewash. First they boil some water, preferably distilled, then they pull apart the capsule and empty the contents into the water and discard the empty capsules. Next they mix the eyebright with the water and allow the water to cool, so that it will not burn the eyes. The water is then strained and poured into an eyecup. The liquid is applied to each eye, and then the treatment is repeated once more. The remaining contents in the pot are then poured into a cup or glass and consumed. The results vary, depending on the severity of the condition.

This is what I told her about eyebright, but before she could answer yes to buying some I mentioned a product called colloidal silver.

"I have just read in Dr. Balch's newest edition of *Prescription for Nutritional Healing* that he recommends colloidal silver as an eyewash for conditions such as yours. If you consider his suggestion, I recommend the Sovereign Silver brand."

I found the page for her and she read what Dr. Balch had written.

"I'll try the silver. How much will I need for the six of us?"

That was on Saturday morning. The following Thursday, another young mother came in with her son. I greeted her and she responded, "Are you Bob?"

"Yes, I am. How can I help you?"

"My friend suggested that I see you about my son. I'm supposed to buy some, some, I think it's called something silver. She said it's good for the eyes. My son has a major problem with dryness. The prescription drops just don't seem to help. I mean they help, but they're not curing the problem, and he can't keep putting drops in his eyes forever. Unless he has to, of course. So I want to buy some of that liquid silver because she said it worked for her entire family."

I asked her what her friend's name was. "It's Hannah. She came in on Saturday to buy some herbs but, at your suggestion, bought the silver instead."

"When you say that it worked for the entire family, to what extent are they better?" I asked.

"All the way better. They used the silver throughout the weekend and the kids went to school on Monday and Anthony went to work. Hannah had to take the kids to school to get them cleared with the school nurse, and they're all okay. When Hannah told me about the silver, I thought it might work for my son's condition."

I asked the mother several questions and, based on her answers, determined that her son was deficient in B-2 and vitamin A. I made her aware of this, but she wanted silver. I showed her some literature that explained the actions and usage of colloidal silver. Then I showed her in Dr. Balch's book the deficiency symptoms of B-2 and vitamin A. This convinced her to go with the vitamins and correct her son's deficiencies, which hopefully would correct the dry-eye problem.

"I hope that this will work for him as well as the silver worked for Hannah's family. Imagine suffering as they did for over three months with their eye conditions, not to mention the money spent and lost because of Anthony's not working. Then they use a God-given mineral—it is a mineral isn't it?—and get better over the weekend. That's a miracle."

She made her purchase of vitamin B-2 and liquid cod liver oil, which was the source for the vitamin A, and said she would keep me aware of her son's progress. Three weeks later she called to tell me that she was pleased beyond belief that the cod liver oil and B-2 had worked so well.

87

Chin Acne

One of my first experiences in identifying deficiencies through body language happened while working for a major vitamin chain in Santa Monica, California, whose store was located just blocks from the Pacific Ocean. This company offered the services of a pharmacy in addition to the vitamin store.

One beautiful Saturday afternoon, a couple walked into the store and ignored my greeting. *Busy,* I thought. The man walked past me and headed directly for the pharmacy section. The woman began checking out the vitamin section. I walked over to her, repeated my greeting, and asked if I could help her find what she was looking for.

She declined my offer by saying she was just looking while her husband shopped. "My husband doesn't believe in vitamins. In his opinion, they are just nonsense and a big money-making racket." With that statement she dismissed me by walking toward our Health and Beauty Aid department.

Grin and bear it, I thought. *She doesn't believe, so why waste my energy on her?* But the dig about our industry, that hurt. I should have walked away, but I sensed that she was still curious about something. I bet it was her face or, more specifically, her chin. During our very brief conversation I noticed the acne, square in the middle of her chin. It was easy to see despite efforts to cover it with makeup. Too much makeup, which actually brought more attention to it. The acne was only on her chin, while the rest of her face was blemish-free. I had to decide whether to ask this non-believer of vitamins a question about the zits on her chin. Why not? That's probably why she went to the Health and Beauty Aid department, to look for a cure.

I walked up to her again and asked if I could ask her a question that might be embarrassing to her. She looked toward her husband and, although he wasn't facing our direction, his closeness assured her that she could call for help if the question was out of line. She nodded okay.

I asked how long she had been afflicted with the acne on her chin.

She instantly put her hand up to her chin as if to try to hide what I had already seen, then answered that it had been a problem for several years. "It's something that comes and goes. I am under the care of an excellent dermatologist."

Perhaps it was the way she had dismissed me earlier, or what she said about her husband's opinion of my industry; I had to go for the dig. "It's too bad your excellent dermatologist doesn't understand the problem." I waited for her to chastise me, but she didn't.

"What do you think the problem is?"

Her question was more a pleading than the sarcasm I was expecting.

I suggested that she stop using (I named a specific brand of toothpaste that was extremely popular in those days).

She countered, "How do you know I use (again mentioning the brand)?"

"Because you have acne on your chin," I answered. I explained to her that many people, women in particular, are sensitive to the fluoride in the toothpaste. It didn't matter how well they rinsed their mouth or how thoroughly they washed their chin after brushing. The fluoride was probably being absorbed through the sublingual glands or just swallowed.

"Your statement that it comes and goes—does that coincide with your menstrual cycle?" I think that, for just a moment, I embarrassed her, as she hesitated before answering. Nevertheless, she nodded yes. I would bet that her excellent dermatologist had never asked her this question.

"Interesting. You must tell my husband what you just said."

I was pleased with her acceptance of my story and hoped her husband would respond with the same attitude.

He had just finished at the pharmacy, so she called him over and asked that he listen to what I had to say. Before I could tell him the story, he said to me that the vitamin industry is just a billion-dollar rip-off and to not talk to him about my racket.

I should have walked away from him, but I didn't. Instead, I corrected him by saying that our industry actually does eight billion dollars a year.

He snickered in contempt.

I continued, "Sir, as big as our industry is, it is still a lot smaller than the donut industry." I turned and started to walk away when his wife called out to me.

"Please tell him what you told me. Please," she pleaded.

Reluctantly, I repeated to him what I had told her.

He put his hand to his chin and said to me, "How interesting. I wonder if I should tell any of my patients or just continue treating them." After finishing his utterance, he turned toward the exit.

I looked at his wife. "Is he the excellent dermatologist who is treating you?"

She quietly answered yes. I then asked what he meant about telling his patients or just continuing to treat them. Her answer almost floored me.

"If he cured his patients of this malady by just advising them to change toothpaste, there would be no income derived from it. That's the decision he has to ponder."

I watched bewildered as she followed her husband. I shook my head in disgust and said a silent prayer for this doctor, who in my opinion was an embarrassment to the human race and to rest of the medical profession.

More stories...

In all these years I have seen many women with acne on the chin, and in every single case the acne disappeared within six weeks.

Once, my wife and I were buying a home and Daryl, the escrow officer, had this same problem. Even the many layers of makeup could not cover her red blemishes. I asked if she would mind my asking her a personal question, and because we were friends she agreed. I suggested that she switch to a fluoride-free toothpaste to correct her problem. She followed my advice and, six weeks later, when we went in to close the escrow, Daryl was proud to show off her blemish-free chin. Six weeks!

A few years ago I thought I had failed a customer named Elizabeth with this advice. She was not a particularly avid vitamin taker but she did indulge in a one-a-day multiple. Without any hesitation, she bought the fluoride-free toothpaste, thanked me for my suggestion, and said she would keep me informed.

About two months later she came into the store. I couldn't help noticing her chin. It was one big red mess of acne. I said apologetically, "Elizabeth, I am sorry, I failed you."

"No, you didn't. I was completely healed just as you said I would be, but last week I went to see my dentist and he said you were wrong. He told me to throw out that other junk toothpaste. He also said that there is no correlation between fluoride and acne. So I took his free sample of fluoride toothpaste, and this is what happened...and all in one week! Please, I need some of yours. I am in a wedding in less than two months and I want to be acne-free.

Note: Will your teeth fall out if you stop using fluoride toothpaste? I don't know. You'll have to ask your dentist. But, remember, the final decision always rests with you. You might want to check the Web and read about all of the atrocities associated with fluoride. Not only in our, no, your toothpaste, but in your drinking water and everywhere else. A nutritional doctor was lecturing on the unhealthful effects of fluoride. He called it "a by-product of aluminum waste."

88

ALLERGIES

'Tis the season—no, not the holiday season—it's allergy season. That stressful, dripping, headachy, hurt-all-over feeling that's both depressing and fatiguing. Interestingly enough, those are just a few symptoms of a deficiency of pantothenic acid, or, as it is uncommonly called, vitamin B-5.

To list the many stories associated with allergies and the overwhelming successes that pantothenic acid has had would fill a book of its own. In her book *Let's Get Well*, Adelle Davis referred to allergies as the pantothenic-acid-deficiency disease.

What was the first word I used above to describe an allergy attack? The word was *stressful*, or *stress*. Whose life is not filled with stress? Most every book on nutrition refers to this vitamin as the "anti-stress pill." Period. I won't go into the many merits of this product; instead, I recommend you refer to Adelle Davis's book or to Dr. Balch's book, *Prescription for Nutritional Healing*.

Countless customers who came into my store asking for something to help in correcting their allergies were always referred to one or both of these books. Why? Because this vitamin works! And, after questioning those who said it didn't work for them, it was determined that they had taken the vitamin just once a day instead of the suggested "throughout the day" indication.

89

Ulcers - Stomach and Duodenal

"Those two young men are huge. I hope you know them. If there ever was a fight, I'd want them to be on my side," my longtime customer said.

"They're a couple of local bodybuilders. I've known them since they were teenagers."

"They look troubled, especially the larger of the two."

I, too, had noticed that they looked as if something was worrying them.

"Well, Bob, I'll leave you so that you can take care of them. Have a good day."

I bade her goodbye and approached the two young men.

"Hey, guys, how are you?"

"Hi, Bob," they answered in unison. The smaller one, who was larger than most men his age, asked if he could use the restroom.

"Of course you can, Les. It's the one with the three letters on the door!" I added jokingly.

When he had gone, I asked his friend Mitch if Les was okay.

Mitch said that Les had been having stomach problems. Maybe it was the flu.

"And how about you, are you feeling okay? You look a little peaked."

"I'm not sick, but my stomach is bothering me. Do you think that, at my age, I could be getting an ulcer? I thought it only happened to older people."

"You could be, although most stomach ulcers occur in people who are middle-aged. Does Les have the same problem as you, or is his the stomach flu?"

"I don't know; neither does he. He probably went to your bathroom to vomit."

"Vomit because he's nauseated, or does he induce vomiting because it takes the pain away?"

When I asked him that, Mitch looked astonished. After a moment, he answered.

"To relieve the pain, but how did you know?"

I didn't answer his question but continued asking mine. "Is he also suffering from bloating or belching, or has he lost his appetite?"

Mitch said that Les did have these symptoms and had been suffering from them for a couple of months. No, Les had not gone to the doctor about this problem. Mitch added that even when Les had lost his appetite, eating usually took the pain away, at least for a few hours, and then the pain would reoccur.

"How about you, Mitch? Do you have the same symptoms as Les?"

"No. I just have burning in my stomach, which sometimes keeps me awake at night. I did call the doctor and he said that he wants to check me out, but that I probably have an ulcer. I've only had this problem for a few days. Can an ulcer happen that fast?"

"Mitch, ulcers have been induced in laboratory animals simply by immobilizing them. This was done by tying the test animals' paws, thus immobilizing the animal overnight. It caused such psychological stress that the animals developed ulcers the next day! Ulcers can be caused by an automobile accident, a severe burn to the body, excess alcohol, or even apprehension because of an impending situation. Yes, ulcers can happen that fast."

Mitch just stood against the counter without saying a word. His hands then went to his stomach.

"Are you hurting, Mitch?"

"Yes, Bob, something awful."

"Can I give you something to drink?" Without waiting for him to answer I went to the back room and reached for a disposable cup, which I filled with aloe vera juice, specifically the brand "George's," which tastes almost like water.

When I returned to the front of the store, Mitch was sitting on the floor, leaning against the wall, and holding his stomach. I offered him the aloe vera.

He took the cup from me and began sipping at the liquid. "I hope I can keep this down. I haven't vomited yet, and I don't want to."

While Mitch continued to sit there, I welcomed another customer and helped her. I kept looking at Mitch to see how he was doing. After several minutes, I finished with my other customer and asked Mitch if he felt any better.

"What kind of water is this? I am feeling better already. This is the first time that drinking water has made my pain go away. Can I have some more?"

I answered yes and took the cup from him, telling him to just stay seated. As I headed to the back room, Les returned from the bathroom, looking very peaked. His face was ashen.

"How about a drink?" I asked.

"No, thanks anyways. I tried drinking some water from the faucet but I couldn't keep it down."

Les walked to the front of the store while I refilled Mitch's cup with the aloe vera juice. This time I returned with the cup plus the bottle of George's aloe.

"I can't believe it, Les, I'm really better. The pain has gone away."

I gave the cup of aloe to Mitch and then showed the two of them the bottle of aloe vera juice.

"This is what you've been drinking. Many of my customers use it to alleviate the pain caused by stomach ulcers. They also use it for external problems such as burns, including sunburn or open wounds. In fact, many people refer to aloe vera juice as 'the miracle plant.'"

"Can I, or should I, be drinking it as well?" asked Les.

"I brought an extra cup for you, but it works faster in Mitch's situation than in yours."

"Why is that? Why wouldn't it work the same?"

"Guys, I'm not a doctor, and I recommend that each of you see one. Mitch, I suspect that you have a stomach ulcer, and, thus, the aloe vera reaches the problem area rather quickly. And you, Les, have symptoms of a duodenal ulcer, which affects the small intestine that leads from the stomach. It takes a lot longer for the aloe to reach that part of the body. Really, guys, as effective as this aloe vera juice is, you both need to get professional medical help, and soon."

"We don't have time to see a doctor. We have things to do first." Les answered as they said their goodbye.

I wondered how two very healthy and health-conscious young men could both develop ulcers, assuming that's what they had.

My assumption was verified just two days later. I read in the local newspaper the cause of their stress. They had apparently been contemplating a robbery of a local retail store, which caused undue stress on their system. They were ultimately arrested and, while incarcerated, were treated medically for their ulcers.

90

Sore Mouth/Tongue

It was an exceptionally busy day for a Tuesday, so I didn't have time to notice this customer's problem until she came to the checkstand. She could barely talk.

"Teeth problems?" I asked.

"No." Her answer was barely audible, but as she spoke I noticed that her tongue was extremely red. It appeared inflamed.

"Are you on any antibiotics?"

She nodded.

"Are you taking them for your sore mouth?"

At first, she appeared agitated by my persistence, but at this last question her eyes opened wider. I had pinpointed her problem.

"No," she mumbled. "I have a, a yeast..." She couldn't finish her sentence because of the pain.

"I know you are hurting, but I want to ask you some more questions. I will ask them so that your answers can be *yes* or *no*. In that way, you don't have to talk, just nod or shake your head. Okay?"

She smiled her thanks and nodded again.

"You have a yeast infection. That's why you're taking antibiotics. Right?"

She nodded.

"How many weeks have you been on antibiotics?" I held up one finger and she shook her head. She had been on antibiotics for four weeks.

"Are you taking any B-complex or a multiple vitamin?"

"No."

"Just shake your head. You don't have to talk, even to say no or yes."

Again, a smile of gratitude.

"Are you taking acidophilus or other milk cultures such as yogurt?"

The look in her eyes told me that she was not familiar with the products I mentioned.

"I'll guess you are not on these products. Is that correct?"

She nodded.

"It's probably very difficult for you to eat with your mouth as sore as it is. Did the doctor put you on any special diet?"

She shook her head.

"Did he say it was okay for you to eat things such as malted milks or milkshakes?"

Her eyes widened and she grinned as she nodded. Apparently she liked her new diet.

"Do your bowel movements have more than the usual odor?" Her face flushed slightly at this question. She nodded and looked toward the floor.

"Any problems with your skin?"

"Like what?"

"Dermatitis, dry skin, itching. Things of that sort."

"Only the itching," she answered hesitantly, still looking at the floor.

"Not on your skin?"

"No. I have other areas that itch."

"Are you being treated for that problem as well?"

"Yes, but to no avail. In fact, it's becoming embarrassingly worse."

"Okay. Let me be candid. Is it vaginal itching?"

"Yes, there too. But that's not the worst area."

"Rectal itching?"

This question caused her to look up at me, more startled than embarrassed.

"Oh my gosh." She was struggling to say the words. "I'm on medicine for that as well as an ointment."

"Do you know whether milk, milk culture, yogurt, or other dairy products are contraindicated for the antibiotics you are taking?"

She nodded, then shook her head no. It must have been the perplexed look on my face that made her smile and painfully say, "Yes, I do know and, no, they are not."

"Are you aware that these additional problems—the sore mouth and tongue and, of course, the itching—are caused by excessive antibiotic intake? This medicine has destroyed your friendly bacteria and probably your B vitamins, too. You've got to restore them in order to get relief."

"Where do I start?"

"Many of my female customers use liquid acidophilus in many ways. Being a liquid, it's more frequently taken orally; however, it can also be applied topically to the areas where there is itching. It can also be added to a douche and/or used as a retention enema."

She gave a sigh as if she now had an answer to her most major problems. She bought some additional B-complex, two bottles of liquid acidophilus, safflower oil capsules, and powdered protein. All of these items would help restore the friendly bacteria that had been destroyed by the excessive use of antibiotics.

I also told her that, because of the high sugar content, those milkshakes, as great tasting as they might be, would only exacerbate her problems.

91

SUGAR WATER

"Good morning, Margaret!" Pat said as the customer walked into the store.

"Hi. Pat, I'd like to introduce you to my friend Denise and her daughter Becky.

"Becky just turned three today, but she's not feeling very well."

"And what's the matter with you, little lady?" asked Pat.

"She has very loose bowels, but she's under doctor's care, so she'll be okay soon." Denise answered for her.

"Denise, she's been sick for a week already! Don't you think that you should get someone else's opinion? At least another doctor's?" Margaret retorted.

Denise didn't respond, but walked to another aisle of the store with her daughter.

Margaret used this opportunity to talk with Pat privately.

"Pat, can you help Becky? I brought them with me so that either you or Bob could give Denise some advice," Margaret pleaded.

"Your friend doesn't seem open to suggestions, Margaret. That always makes it almost impossible to render advice. I'll try. Tell me, what was the doctor's diagnosis?"

"Just loose bowels. No fever or any other symptoms. He didn't even call it a stomach flu—just diarrhea, probably caused by something in the air. Whatever that means."

"Does Becky have problems keeping food down?"

"I don't know." She called out to her friend, "Denise, whether you like it or not, I've been discussing Becky's problem with Pat. Does Becky have any trouble eating?"

With a somewhat disgusted look on her face Denise answered abruptly, "She wasn't eating much anyway, so the doctor told me to just put her on sugar water. She drinks that without any problem."

"Has she been getting any better, or is she worse since drinking the sugar water?" Pat asked.

It was Margaret who answered. "As far as I'm concerned, she's been getting worse the last few days. Denise, don't you agree?"

"Look. I'm no doctor, and this is my first child, so I don't have any experience in these matters. I can only trust that the doctor knows what he's doing. After all, he is the professional." She hesitated a moment, then added, "Pat, I'm sorry, I didn't mean that as an insult to you. I meant that he, oh never mind. Pat, what can I do for Becky?"

"Denise, we have never suggested to anyone to stop taking what was prescribed by the doctor. No exceptions. If you ask me what I would do if Becky were my child, that I can tell you. Then the decision is up to you."

"What would you do?" asked Denise.

"Instead of sugar and water, you might consider sugar and milk. That would give Becky some lactose, which does support friendly bacteria. I personally would give my children acidophilus in liquid form. I have it in both plain and strawberry flavor." Pat didn't say any more; her silence gave Denise time to reach a personal decision.

"I'll go with the plain."

That was Thursday.

Friday afternoon, Denise called and left a message for Pat. "Becky is all better, thanks to you and the acidophilus."

On Saturday morning, Denise called and told Pat that Becky had a recurrence of diarrhea and added, "Your acidophilus stopped working. I had to put Becky back on the sugar water."

"Denise, you left a message for me yesterday saying that Becky was all better. Did you stop giving her the acidophilus at that time?"

"Yes. I thought she was well, so I stopped giving it to her."

For several moments, Pat did not answer. Finally, Denise broke the silence. "Pat, I goofed, didn't I? I'll start Becky on the acidophilus immediately."

On Monday afternoon, a young mother came in and asked for Pat, who was not at the store at that moment.

"Tell her that I'm going to pick up some acidophilus for my four-year-old little boy. He has diarrhea, and I was told by my neighbor to get it to correct his problem. My neighbor said she was in here on Thursday and that's what she bought for her daughter and it worked. She also told me to make sure I continue giving it to him and not stop, even though he might appear to get better the next day. In fact, she asked that I buy a bottle for her as well."

92

WHAT ARE YOUR FEARS?

I can relate to those who fear things. My fear was driving my car. I had reached the point where I thought it was time to turn in my driver's license and give the car keys to my wife.

My first attack occurred while I was driving home late at night from Laughlin, Nevada. I tried passing an eighteen-wheeler that was traveling about sixty miles per hour. I pulled alongside, and that's as far as I got. In my mind I had visions of crashing, so I backed off and trailed the truck for a few miles. It was a strange feeling, as passing had never been a problem before. I thought that maybe my windshield was dirty; I blamed it on my new eyeglasses; perhaps it was because it was so late and I was more tired than I thought. I tried passing once more, and again I backed off because of the fear of crashing. That was my first episode with this problem.

Traveling on the surface streets was no problem, just driving the freeway. It didn't matter if it was day or night—the problem persisted. Driving on a straightaway wasn't the problem—it was when I had to negotiate a curve in the roadway or passing. I knew that the speed limit was 65mph and that most curves, unless marked differently, could be safely driven at double the speed limit. I knew that, yet I slowed down to an unsafe 45mph. I became a hazard to other drivers. I contemplated giving up driving on the freeways.

That's when I was introduced to a Bach Flower remedy called mimilus. My first experience with mimilus was in Alabama. My wife and I had just flown there for an eventual vacation in Florida, which ultimately meant a few hours of driving. I placed five drops of the flower remedy under my tongue, per the instructions, and got on the freeway. I was a little apprehensive when I came upon my first curve in the roadway. I started to reduce my speed, but since there were no other cars behind me I continued into the curve at the speed limit. I made it! I was so excited I took another five drops under my tongue, as directed. That's all it took, one bottle of this amazing flower remedy, and I was cured. I used the mimilus for about a year, and that was over seven years ago. Now I jokingly say to drivers who have similar fears, "Take your mimilus!"

The indication for taking mimilus is for known fears. How many of you have a fear of flying, elevators, the dentist, amusement park rides, riding a bicycle, heights, or driving your automobile on the freeway? After I learned its effectiveness, this product helped many of my customers.

93

TOOTHACHE

How can you see a toothache? You can't. But you can see the suffering associated with having one.

I was at the bank preparing a deposit when I saw this couple enter. She got in line behind me while he stood at the door.

I'm always looking for things in people. Their hair, their eyes, the way they stand or walk, scars, acne, or if they have a cold or are sneezing. It's just me— when I see someone apparently suffering, I have to ask why or how.

Of this couple, I noticed that the man had a problem. The side of his face looked inflamed and slightly swollen. So I asked the woman if he had a toothache, and she answered that he did.

"I hope he has a good dentist," was my reply.

She answered that they did; in fact, it was her brother, but he was out of town. So they had to make an appointment with another dentist.

She continued, "This dentist required a check for a hundred dollars, whereas with my brother it would have been free." She sighed that they had no choice.

I answered, "Yes, you did. And, if you don't mind waiting, I'll explain after I make my deposit."

She said she would wait, and I moved to the teller to do my banking.

Upon completion of my deposit, I saw that the couple was waiting for me at the counter. I approached them but did not introduce myself, as I was about to prescribe something to remedy his pain. At the store I would have used stories as references in order to avoid prescribing, but he was hurting and I wanted to speed things up.

I told them he would need a Waterpik or similar device.

They had one.

Next, they should go to a vitamin store and purchase a product called GSE, made by the Nutribiotics Company. Put fifteen drops in the container, add warm water, set the control of the spray at two or three, and direct the solution directly into the problem area. I emphasized that they should limit the amount of GSE to fifteen drops, as more could irritate the gum. I knew what his next question would be, so I told him that he should have relief within the hour and to repeat the procedure as necessary.

The next day I found out that the vitamin store this couple had chosen was mine! My employees had confirmed my suggestion of the GSE, and they gave them literature reassuring them that it would work. And it did.

They called the store just two hours later, telling my employee that the extract had worked so well and so fast that they cancelled the appointment with the dentist. They felt comfortable enough about GSE that they would wait until the woman's brother returned home in two days.

GSE, or grapefruit seed extract, is an amazing gift from Nature. I have countless stories as to its effectiveness, not only for toothaches, but for gingivitis as well. It is not a replacement for professional help, but it does work well in an emergency.

94

Green Tea

This story does not have anything to do with a nutritional deficiency, but it is about something that affects most everyone at some time, regardless of age. That something is a sore. And more specifically, a sore within the mouth. Ouch, such pain! And the tongue, that inquisitive tongue! It always seems to be searching for something, whether it's that sore spot, the hole in a tooth, a brand-new filling, recent gum surgery, or the canker sore on the side of the cheek. And when it finds and touches the hurting area, it usually intensifies the pain.

This customer was allowing his wife to do the shopping while he stood in the corner next to the book display. He was holding a handkerchief next to his mouth. I sidled over to ask him if I could help him find what he might be looking for. Before turning to answer me, he placed in his mouth what he had been holding in his handkerchief. It was his dentures. I could only surmise that he had a problem with them. If you've read this far in this book, you realize that I of course had to satisfy my nosey curiosity. Before he could answer my first question, I asked him another. Were his dentures ill-fitting, or did he have a sore in his mouth? His answer confirmed that he had what is the bane of many denture wearers—a mouth sore. Being a denture wearer myself and having gone through the intensive and painful surgeries, I could relate to his problem. I told him about green tea and its propensity to heal.

I, too, initially learned about green tea from another denture wearer, who was also my customer. He saw me hurting at the store one day and was bold enough to ask if I wore dentures and, if so, was that what was causing my pain. He told me how he used green tea to relieve the pain of mouth sores and how it promoted the healing process. He boiled some water, poured it into a cup along with a green tea bag and some honey. After drinking the tea, he removed his dentures and placed the tea bag in his mouth, directly onto the area of the sore. His tongue, that curious tongue, could then hold the tea bag on the sore for as long as possible. Preferably for an hour or more! I decided to follow his instructions explicitly, except that I held the bag against the sore area with my tongue for two hours, while working on the computer. I could not believe how the pain lessened in that short time. I repeated the process the next morning while showering and dressing for work. My sore mouth was no longer sore. The green tea had worked almost miraculously.

I have conveyed this story to countless denture wearers, to my personal dentist, and to the dentists who are my customers. If you are bothered with any of the problems associated with mouth sores, do yourself a healing favor and follow the instructions of my bold customer.

The green tea story doesn't end with mouth sores. A first-time customer came rushing into my store early one morning. She was holding a baggie filled with ice up to her eye.

"Where's the tea section?" she asked. "I need some green tea bags."

Because of my past episode with green tea and a sore mouth, I believed that I knew the reason for her request. She, too, knew the healing properties of green tea. She told me that after going to work that morning, a female co-worker had accidentally hit her in the eye with her elbow.

"I have a first date tonight and I don't want to have a black eye."

Seeing the damage when she lowered the ice-filled baggie from her eye, I thought the application of a green tea bag would be too late to fix the problem. Her eye was red and swollen, as was the area beneath her eye, and was already turning black-and-blue. The young lady came in the following day just to show me her eye, her healed eye. She said that the discoloring had lessened to the point were it required only a minimal amount of cosmetic powder to cover the injured area prior to going out with her new date. Smiling, she added that the date had gone well.

These are just two of the many stories extolling the merits of green tea. Others have used it on sores and even lesser open wounds anywhere and everywhere on the body. One customer, whose dog was in a fight with a cat, taped a tea bag on the scratched area of the dog's ear.

95

PINWORMS

"Ma'am, did you know that you are being followed?" I asked my customer as she entered the store.

First she looked at me as if trying to comprehend what I had just said. Then she looked behind her and smiled. "Oh, that little guy. He's my protector. He follows me everywhere," she said fondly of her son. She then introduced him to me.

"Greg, this is Bob. Bob, this is my son, Greg. He's my protector. My little follower."

I extended my hand to her son, and, for a young boy of about seven, he had a good grip. I did note, however, that, although his hand was not the least bit cold, it was moist—almost too moist. I wondered if the moistness was caused by too much sugar in his diet or a blood sugar problem. My curiosity would prompt me to find out. Nosey me. The boy also seemed too thin and too pale for this time of year. So much for my initial assessment of Greg; then I decided to turn my attention to his mom and find out if her hands were moist as well.

"Joyce," I said, extending my hand to hers, "you have a fine young man in Greg. You should be proud. How old is he?" I had determined that her hand was neither moist nor cold. Why was Greg's? Was this inherited from his dad?

"Greg is just a few months shy of nine," she said.

I was somewhat taken aback when I heard his age; he looked so much younger.

"Greg, Bob has some books and toys for you to play with while I do my shopping. I'll be just a short while."

As Joyce and I discussed her vitamin purchase, I kept looking over at her son and wondering if he had a problem or if it was just my imagination. It wasn't until about five minutes into our conversation that I noticed Greg was scratching at his bottom. *Just an itch,* I thought. I continued my conversation with his mother, and, a few minutes later, Greg repeated his scratching. Hmmm. Moist hands, pale, thin, small in stature, and possible rectal itching.

I whispered to Joyce, "I noticed that Greg is scratching his bottom. Does he have a bug bite?"

"No, no bug bite—just a bad habit. We've been trying to stop him from doing it, and he promises to stop, but, if you noticed it, I guess he hasn't."

"Have you had him checked by his pediatrician?"

"No. Why? Just for a bad habit?"

"Maybe it's more than a habit. Have you considered that it might be pinworms?"

"Bob, I'm sorry, but that's disgusting!" With that statement she turned from me and proceeded to the other side of the store. I stood there helpless, wondering what to do. She was adamant in not wanting to discuss the possibility of worms, and yet what if Greg did have them? There were just too many symptoms pointing in that direction. I had to persist.

"Joyce, it's apparent that I owe you an apology for bringing up such a subject. As you know, sometimes I get curious."

"Maybe too curious at times" was her abrupt answer as she moved to the checkout counter.

I silently rang up her purchase on the register, but my mind was racing. How could I bring the subject up again without annoying her further? Fortunately, she broke the silence.

"What made you ask that question?" she asked. Her voice was somewhat apologetic.

"Which one? I asked so many." I asked. Did she realize that I was bantering with her?

She smiled and answered, "You know, the disgusting one."

"Joyce," I started, "when Greg and I shook hands I noticed that his hand was moist. That was my first clue. Next, he's somewhat small in stature, probably smaller than others his age."

The nodding of her head indicated that she agreed, but she still did not answer.

"Greg is a little on the pale side, and this is June. Where is his suntan? Doesn't he like the sun or doesn't he tan readily?"

"He's pale," she said quietly as she looked toward the floor rather than at me. "I mentioned it to my husband, but he said that Greg is just spending too much time inside the house. That's not true, but my husband didn't want to hear that, so I just agreed with him and said I would force Greg outside more often. I know you're not a doctor, but I also know you have some ideas. Go ahead, ask me what you need to know."

"Just one more question. What are Greg's favorite foods?"

"All he eats is sugar. Cookies, cake, bread, pasta, and candy if my husband brings it home. He absolutely won't eat meat or eggs, and he pushes his vegetables away as well. I don't know what to do anymore. He's skinny as a rail, I know, but I'm not getting any help from my husband!"

"Joyce, I suspect pinworms, especially with the diet Greg has—all sugar. Worms and parasites love that kind of diet. In fact, parasites thrive on sugar. He needs his protein and veggies, of course, but he also needs lots of the B vitamins and vitamin A. You might also consider acidophilus or yogurt. I have read in many articles by herbalists that garlic is the herb of choice in cleansing the intestines of parasites and worms. In fact, many animal owners use garlic to de-worm their dogs, especially the puppies."

"Where do I start?" she asked pleadingly.

"First, you must convince your husband that Greg probably has a parasite problem. Next, make an appointment with the pediatrician. Greg needs professional help."

"What if the doctor finds that he has worms? What do they do for that?"

"If he does have a parasitic problem, the doctors will probably give him antihelmintic drugs, which either kill or paralyze the worms. This is followed by a laxative to expel the worms from the body. It's a simple process."

"Bob, I believe that I'm a very good housekeeper, how could he have gotten worms, that is, if he does have them?"

"Eating raw fish is one example."

"We don't do that."

"Maybe from contact with infected soil or water. Do you do any camping?"

"Oh my gosh. We went on vacation at my aunt's home back East. They have a duck pond in their backyard, and we caught Greg and his cousins wading in the water. Could this have been the cause?"

"Yes, especially if he swallowed some of the water. Were they doing more than wading?"

"Greg, when we were at Aunt Gussie's this year, besides wading did you and your cousins swim in the duck pond? Greg, I really need to know."

"Yes. When we were chasing the ducks and geese, we fell in. Then we just played in the water for awhile."

"That, Joyce, could be the explanation if he has a parasite problem. At this point, it's all conjecture until you find out from the doctor. But first, you've got to convince your husband."

Joyce thanked me for the information I had given her, and then she and Greg said goodbye and left the store. She called the next day to say that her husband thought the worm idea was a bunch of hooey. I suggested she have a long talk with her son and be specific in her questioning about why Greg needs to scratch his bottom end. She called me a couple of hours later, crying. Greg had told her that it felt like something was crawling around his bottom end, which made him want to scratch at it.

"Bob, I feel so terrible about the way I scolded Greg for what I thought was a bad habit. I can't forgive myself. I'm going to have Greg tell his father what he just told me. Maybe that will convince my husband that Greg does have a parasite problem and needs professional help."

It was determined that Greg had pinworms. The appropriate drugs were administered, and over the next few months Greg improved dramatically. He even began enjoying his veggies.

96

Being Overweight - A Deficiency of

Perhaps one of the most obvious symptoms of a nutritional deficiency is being overweight. Unfortunately, what that deficiency may be has not been determined. Through the years, several theories have circulated concerning the correlation between nutrition and weight, but no one theory has been found to be the answer. A few dieters have been fortunate enough to lose weight, about 3 percent, but the majority of those who lose weight gain it back.

When I had been in this industry one year, the liquid protein diet was introduced into the marketplace. Literally tens of thousands of people lost a combined total of hundreds of thousands, if not millions, of pounds on this program. But it was an impossible diet to maintain, and most of the lost weight was eventually gained back. I, too, sold the liquid protein diet to my customers, hoping that this product would help them lose weight as advertised. Today, I apologize for my naivete. After the popularity of the liquid protein diet ran its course, the Cambridge diet was introduced. Again, I apologize for promoting it. I should also apologize for promoting the many diets that followed, year after year, because I truly believed that one of them just might work.

In the late1970s I decided there wasn't a magic pill or, for that matter, a magic protein powder for weight loss. Even though I continued selling the next new generation of diet programs, I did not actively promote them. In my mind I knew that these diets wouldn't work. About that time I developed my own theory about weight loss. However, I referred to it as fat loss. From that point on, I tried selling customers on my theory, a fat-loss program, in addition to the newest diet fad.

Miranda was the first customer to consider trying my non-diet. She was about fifty pounds overweight and suffered from diabetes. She had tried numerous diets with no success. On an eventful Monday evening, at least for me, Miranda, amongst others, listened to my lecture, but it was only she who actually bought the supplements I had recommended. These included lecithin capsules, safflower oil capsules, and a protein powder. I also gave specific instructions as to how to balance the amounts of fats, proteins, and carbohydrates in what you eat. I called it "proportional eating."

Miranda called me the next day at one-thirty. I could hear her trepidation as she said, with a quavering voice, "Your diet doesn't work for me. I'm having a diabetic attack."

Mentally I reviewed my suggestion for her breakfast: a poached egg, some cottage cheese, a couple of prunes, and enough liquid to swallow her supplements. *A perfect breakfast,* I thought, *certainly enough of the correct foods to last the four to five hours necessary to maintain her blood sugar level.*

"Miranda, what did you have for breakfast?"

"Just what you told me to have. It was delicious. I really enjoyed it, but apparently it doesn't work for me."

"And you took the supplements?"

"Yes, although they were a lot to swallow."

Everything seemed correct—proportional amounts of protein, carbohydrates, and fat, along with the friendly fats in the supplements. I was perplexed.

"Miranda, what time did you eat breakfast?"

She didn't answer. I waited for what seemed like several minutes, but was really a few seconds. She still didn't answer.

"Miranda? Are you okay?"

She finally answered. "Bob!" Again, there was silence. Another eternity passed before she responded. "Bob, I have complete control of my life!"

I could hear her sobbing.

She repeated her statement. "Bob, I can't believe it. I can control my life, even control my diabetes, instead of it controlling me."

I liked what I heard her say, but I didn't know what she meant.

She finally filled me in. "Bob, I ate breakfast at eight o'clock this morning. I went without food for almost six hours! I've never been able to do that before. If I had eaten lunch when you suggested, after four or five hours at the most, I wouldn't be having this blood sugar attack. I waited too long to eat, but that's great, because now, because of what you told me last night, now I can control my blood sugar with proper and timely eating."

Whew! I don't have the space in this book to relate all of what was going through my mind in the few seconds before she explained her realization.

Miranda continued eating this proportioned way for the next several weeks. She even was exercising, although this meant walking around the block twice. But it was more than she had ever done before, because of the pain it had caused in her legs due to the diabetes.

Because of Miranda's success, my enthusiasm grew and I continued promoting my theory of proportional eating to customers who were pursuing a weight-loss program. Unfortunately, only a very few ever heeded my advice, and, because there wasn't any scientific proof to my theory, many listened to their friends and others who convinced them that my theory was crazy. After all, why would someone want to put more fat into their diet when that was what they were trying to lose? How could I convince anyone that my theory was correct? This was in 1980.

It was up to me to write a book about fat loss! What better way to promote an idea to the masses than through a book? Based on the successes, although limited, of the continually arriving new weight-loss programs, I could see that people believed authors. Even before starting my first book, I sent letters to several publishers to see if there would be an interest. I was amazed when two publishers responded that they were indeed interested in my book proposal. Perhaps it was the title, *Eat Fat, to Lose Fat!*, that caught their interest. What an attention-getter! In my mind I could see the headlines blasted on the front page of the grocery store tabloids. VITAMIN STORE OWNER SOLVES THE MYSTERY OF FAT LOSS! EAT FAT TO LOSE FAT.

I needed help to do the necessary research for a 300-page book. Three hundred pages? Perhaps it was the number, *300*, that was my first stumbling block. Next, and probably the most daunting, was the fact that most everyone in my industry thought the idea was crazy. How could introducing more fat into the diet actually make people lose weight? Again, this was 1980. I was defeated. I did what those I wanted to help did: I gave up.

A few years later, in 1986, a book by Udo Erasmus was published. It was titled *Fats and Oils*. This well-written book, which contains many documented studies, proved to me that my theory had been correct, but by then my enthusiasm for writing my own book had dwindled. Several years later, another book, this one by Dr. Barry Sears, was introduced. It was titled *Enter the Zone*. Again, that which I had been preaching for years was now in print.

Although I didn't write my own book, I started on the lecture circuit once more. Now I had the proof, backed by two very learned authors, to validate my fat-loss theory. I, too, needed to lose some fat, about fifteen pounds' worth, as well as a couple of inches around the middle. I became an enthusiastic follower of my own program. After just a couple of weeks, I was experiencing great progress. Unfortunately, I had a friend who followed me wherever I went. I couldn't shake him, and he was trying to convince me that I was doing the wrong thing.

He would be there when I ate lunch and dinner. I couldn't even shake him when I had my breakfast. He would shadow me at parties or at friends' homes, especially when they were serving snacks. He even tried taking walks with me or participating in my morning sit-up exercises. He was everywhere.

He actually encouraged me to eat that extra slice of toast at breakfast, to have a malted milk for lunch or ice cream at night before going to bed. He would tell me, "It's okay to cheat a little." It became apparent that he was trying to discourage me from partaking in my own program. At parties he convinced me to eat the fattening snacks that were being offered. And why should I have to get up so early in the morning to go for a walk? It was just too cold outside! Or was it too hot? Either way, he did his best to talk me out of walking and, in particular, out of doing sit-ups. "Do you want to hurt your back?" he would ask. I knew what I needed to do, follow the program to lose unwanted fat in order to maintain my health, but he convinced me otherwise. And he won.

Who was this other person?

He was me! The other guy, the other me, who so convincingly talked me out of my program. He's the culprit. I'm convinced that it is the other person in each of us who suggests that it's okay to cheat just once, or maybe twice, or... He or she doesn't want us to look thin because he or she is the fat person within us. And to him, being fat is comfortable.

Okay, this is just another theory of mine.

But this theory evolved into another theory. Weight loss is a deficiency, after all! And now, I understand what the deficiency is! It affected me while I was trying to lose weight, and it affected me when I was trying to write my first book. I believe it affects others who are trying to diet—and not just dieting. This deficiency affects people who try to accomplish other things as well, causing them to either fail in their endeavors or stop pursuing them. I believe that we are all deficient in the same thing! It's discipline! Think about it. We mean well in our endeavors, but isn't the road to failure paved with good intentions?

97

Breast Cysts

"Hi, Bob. Happy Saturday," said the customer who had just entered my store. I smiled at her. "Gotcha!" she said and then continued. "It's always you who says the happy whatever day it is to us."

"Good morning Mrs. Smyth. How may I help you?"

"I'm not here to buy anything. I just came in for a hug, a celebration hug," she answered, approaching me with open arms. As I returned the hug she continued, "This is more than a hug, Bob, this is my double-breasted hug."

Several customers were already in the store when Mrs. Smyth came in. Sharing hugs in the store was never a big deal, in fact, we did it all the time, but this situation was different. The "double-breasted" phrase got everyone's attention. I looked at Mrs. Smyth, saw the happy grin on her face, and asked if she would like to explain what she meant.

Proudly, she said aloud, "Yesterday, I was told by my oncologist that I no longer have cysts in my breasts and, consequently, it is no longer necessary for me to undergo a double mastectomy as was proposed a few months ago. Bob gave me the encouragement to try some alternative measures—not instead of, but in addition to, allopathic medicine. I did, and now I am still a whole woman."

Mrs. Smyth had come into my store several months earlier as a referral customer. After we exchanged greetings, I asked what I could help her with, in addition to the chapping above her upper lip.

She reached for her nose and said, "Oh, this? No, this is caused by my allergies. I'm here about the stress in my life. I was hoping there might be a substitute for the medicine I am currently taking."

"What are you doing for your allergies? Are you on any medication for that problem?"

"Yes and no. What the doctor prescribed makes me so sleepy, I can hardly function. Especially driving. I stopped taking it except on weekends, such as today. I can live with the allergies; it's the stress I need help with."

"There might be a correlation between the two. Why are you so stressed-out?"

"I'm supposed to get married in a few months."

"That's a good reason to be stressed."

"Bob, I'm fifty years old. I have been divorced for several years now and never planned on remarrying until, until he came along. I fell in love all over again! It was strange, going out on our first date. I didn't know how to act or what to expect. After a few weeks, I, we found the lumps in my breasts. I panicked! When I was in my early twenties I had ovarian cancer, which was subsequently cured through surgery and the usual medication. But now, would I be able to go through it all over again?"

"You went to the doctor, of course?"

"Yes. I was told that I should undergo a double mastectomy. They wanted to remove both of my breasts, which would, in my opinion, make me a less-than-whole woman for my husband-to-be. Yes, we both fell in love and are planning a typical June wedding. Isn't that enough to be stressed-out about?"

"Let's talk about your allergies."

"Why do you keep asking me about my allergies? It's the thought of losing my breasts, or my life, that I'm concerned about," she said somewhat disgusted with my continued questioning about her allergies.

"As I said earlier, there could be a correlation. Would you mind answering a few questions for me on this questionnaire?"

I handed her the Body Language Questionnaire, and she briefed through the pages.

"A few? There's almost three hundred!"

"Most of those you can do at home. I just need for you to answer a few to see if my hunches are correct."

I explained that stress could weaken the adrenal glands, which could also affect the immune system, thus lessening her chances of correcting her ills—whatever they might be. Her answers to my questions convinced her to purchase a B-complex, a multi-mineral formula, and pantothenic acid. Additionally, I gave her literature with respect to taking vitamin E to dissolve breast cysts. (This was in the early 1990s, before the introduction of hormonal creams.)

"I'll buy the vitamin E today because I know that the literature you gave me will convince me to try it."

Mrs. Smyth read the literature and, based on that and with the cooperation of her doctor, eventually increased her daily intake of this vitamin to 1,600 units. Over the next few months, I knew she had controlled the stress in her life. Even her chapped upper lip cleared up, and she was happy about her impending marriage. But it wasn't until that Happy Saturday that I learned about her clean bill of health and her not needing the double mastectomy.

98

Fibrositis

Fibrositis is not an affliction most people are aware of. In fact, most doctors don't accept it as an illness, and the word *fibrositis* is not a medical term. Nevertheless, Tia was diagnosed with this problem. At first, because of the symptoms, she thought she had arthritis. She suffered from pain and stiffness in her back, legs, knees, and shoulders.

"No," she was told by one doctor. "Most doctors diagnose your symptoms as arthritis, but that's because, unfortunately, they're not familiar with fibrositis. I'll give you a mild painkiller, but have your husband massage your muscles around your joints as well as your back." That was the treatment of choice. Nothing for curing the problem, only painkillers for relief.

I didn't know Tia, except by name. She was a friend of my wife, and one evening we joined her and her husband, Mike, for dinner. Upon being introduced

I shook her hand, checking for coldness or moistness, then focused on her fingers, specifically her ring fingers. They had what many women refer to as "the tarnished look." I also noted that her shoulders were slumped, nor did she stand tall or sit tall in her chair. It appeared to me that Tia had several mineral deficiencies, but I didn't make any comment to anyone, including my wife, Pat. When the main course was served, Tia asked her husband if she could have the lemon from his iced tea. He obliged her. She squeezed the lemon over her entree, tasted the food, and then asked Pat for her lemon. Nothing wrong with adding lemon to fish, but Tia had ordered chicken. Apparently, Pat's lemon wasn't enough to satisfy Tia. She asked the waiter for more lemons and, upon his return, promptly used most of them. Again, I didn't make any comment.

It was during the small talk that occurs after dinner that I first learned of the condition called fibrositis.

"My doctor said there isn't a cure, so I have Mike massage my back whenever I'm in pain."

The look on Mike's face revealed that this was a less-than-pleasurable task. I got the feeling that Tia liked the attention and, thus, didn't mind the pain.

I couldn't help myself, "Do you always add lemon to chicken?"

"It gives it a better taste," said Tia in a matter-of-fact tone.

I continued, "Did the doctor ever check your pH balance?" I saw a look of uncertainty in Tia's expression, so I explained what "pH" meant.

"Oh, I'm sure my doctor checked for that. He's very good. After all, it was he, and only he, who discovered my problem." *Case closed*, I thought.

A few weeks later we joined Mike and Tia, along with others, at a local community event. One of the concession stands was selling pickles.

"Mike, buy me a pickle, the largest they have!" said Tia to her husband.

She was the only one within our group who indulged in eating a pickle. I tucked that information away in my brain, but I decided to talk to Mike about his wife and her condition. After questioning him in an indirect fashion I learned that, besides having fibrositis, Tia also suffered from leg cramps, menstrual cramping, and severe dental problems. These are additional symptoms of a deficiency of minerals, specifically calcium and magnesium. I also suspected a deficiency of enzymes, particularly hydrochloric acid. Later that evening, I discussed my thoughts about Tia with my wife.

"Honey," I asked, "how do I approach her with this information, or is the job up to you?"

"Bob," said my realistic wife, "you've already approached her once, and she shot you down. Perhaps she doesn't want to get better; after all, her affliction is not life-threatening, and she obviously enjoys the attention she receives, especially from her husband."

Pat was correct in her thinking, but instead of closing the case I put it on hold. Maybe, at sometime in the future, Tia would ask about pH balance.

It took two weeks before the opportunity came about. Pat and I were at a friend's home for a patio party. We were at the appetizer table when Mike and Tia joined us. Tia zeroed in on the pickles and cherry tomatoes, putting several of each on her plate. Within minutes, she consumed at least seven or eight tomatoes. Even Pat noticed how many Tia had eaten.

"Oh, I just love these cherry tomatoes," said Tia, "I could eat a whole bowlful."

Since it was just the four of us—Tia and Mike, Pat and me—I said, "Tia, a few weeks ago, I mentioned that I suspected you might have a pH imbalance. Your body appears to be out of balance, pH-wise."

"Bob, you're not going to start that thing again, are you?" she asked.

"I'm just going to mention it once more, that's all. Please, give me just a couple of minutes to state my case." I didn't wait for her approval, or disapproval.

"Tia, you eat tomatoes, pickles, and use lemon more than the usual."

"It's because I like them. It has nothing to do with my condition."

"Allow me the two minutes, please, then I will never mention it again, unless, of course, you want to discuss it with me. These are just some symptoms of a deficiency of minerals: leg cramps, difficulty falling asleep, poor posture, slumping of the shoulders, joint pain, and dental problems."

"Except for the joint pain, I don't have any of those, what you call 'deficiency symptoms,'" she said looking, no glaring, at Mike. He turned away.

I continued, "If a person doesn't have enough stomach acid, specifically hydrochloric acid, he or she is not able to assimilate minerals. Because of your eating habits, I suspect you have a system that is out of balance, and you really should have your doctor do a pH test, both on your blood and your urine."

Tia turned to look at Pat. "Does he always insult your friends this way?"

In my defense Pat answered, "He's only trying to help. Please consider what he is saying."

Mike joined in. "Be honest with yourself, and to all of us here. Bob has pegged your problems, and yet you want to ignore them. Listen! Just once, listen to what you are being told. Wouldn't it be nice to mend those problems just by correcting your mineral deficiencies?"

"It's time for us to leave this affair. Parties are supposed to be for fun, not to be embarrassed," said Tia as she turned and proceeded to the front door.

"Pat, Bob. I am so sorry. She just won't admit the truth. I don't know what to do anymore." With that, Mike hugged Pat goodbye, patted me on the shoulder, and thanked us both for trying.

Several weeks later, in a very apologetic tone of voice, Tia called to invite us over for iced tea and dessert. She had finally accepted that she had lots of problems. She also asked if we knew of a different doctor, one who would recognize her problems and treat them accordingly.

While my customers readily accepted my suggestions, friends and relatives were more often difficult to convince.

99

Shingles

"Hi, Doris. Happy Friday."

"Hi, Bob, and a Happy Friday to you too. Bob, this is my father, Ted. He's going to stay with me and my family for awhile, at least until he's comfortable living by himself."

"I lost my wife," said Ted sadly. "We had been married for over forty years, and now she's gone."

I offered my hand for him to shake. I needed to determine some basis for any deficiencies he might have. He had a good grip, his hand was reasonably warm, and there was no noticeable moisture on the palm, but I did notice him twinge slightly as I touched his shoulder with my other hand. The usual illnesses ran through my mind as to the cause of the obvious irritation I induced by touching. Bad shoulder, sunburn, injury, or could it just be caused by the undue stress he has over the loss of his wife? That's when I saw the rash on his upper arm.

Doris interrupted my thoughts, "Dad has been under a lot of stress. He also has a lingering cold, and his hay fever has surfaced again. I brought him here to take the deficiency questionnaire."

"Ted, what medications are you on?"

"Just cortisone, and some kind of salve."

"Did you ever have chicken pox?"

"Doesn't everybody get that?" asked Doris.

"Ted?" I asked it as a question.

"Yeah, I had that too."

"Are you taking the cortisone for the hay fever, or for your shingles?"

"For the hay fever, but, how did you know I have shingles?"

"An educated guess. When I touched your arm you flinched, so I looked for a possible cause and saw the rash on your arm. Are the shingles just on your arm, or on your abdomen as well?"

"Across the left side of my chest, under my arm, and on top of my shoulder, exactly where you touched."

"The salve, is that what was prescribed for the shingles?"

"Yes, but it's not working."

Again, Doris responded, "He's been suffering from these shingles for almost eight months. They started in April. Right, Dad? Or was it May?"

"June. It was late June, just before your mother passed on. It was early April when the hay fever started."

"Ted, have you been on cortisone since April?"

"Yeah, according to the doctor, it's the treatment of choice."

"Ted, Doris. I think the two of you should have a long talk with the doctor. Shingles has several causes, including chicken pox."

Ted interrupted me, "But I had that almost sixty years ago."

"But it never goes away."

"What?" asked Ted and Doris, almost in unison.

"Once you get chicken pox, it never really goes away. It, actually the chicken pox virus, stays hidden in the body, sometimes forever, without ever causing a problem. Ted, you've been under a lot of stress. You probably have a weakened immune system, indicated by your inability to rid yourself of the cold. And, excessive cortisone could exasperate the problem. Together, these factors could have caused the virus to be activated, but instead of chicken pox it became shingles!"

"Well the symptoms are the same. Pain, itching, rash, and blisters. Do you have any suggestions?" asked Ted.

"Bob, I think you convinced Dad to do the questionnaire," said Doris. "Is there something that can be done nutritionally, as well as medically?"

"Doris, I think that we will find your dad very deficient in all of the B vitamins, but especially B-1. A specific deficiency of this vitamin is skin sensitivity. I've heard of many success stories with this vitamin for this very condition. Additionally, the book *Prescription for Nutritional Healing* recommends the amino acid L-lysine as well as the vitamins A, C, pantothenic acid, and... Here you two, read the book yourselves."

100

CHOOSING A DOCTOR

Throughout the years, I was asked, "What doctor can you recommend?" Or, "How do I go about finding a good doctor?"

The answer was simple. "Ask a nurse! Find out who she, or he, goes to." I say that, but with reservations.

If you ask a nurse who works at a doctor's office, he or she will likely suggest that doctor. After all, if he or she didn't, it could possibly affect his or her job.

I always recommend that a person go to a hospital and spend a few hours in the cafeteria. Those are the nurses to ask! They work for the hospital, not for a specific doctor, and, because they see the doctors in action, they are able to determine the doctors' abilities and, very importantly, their bedside manners. Does the doctor care, or is the patient just another body?

Because I don't mind hospital food, this practice is easy for me. That's how we chose our doctor, and I compliment and thank the many nurses who suggested him.

101

HOPEFULLY, A HAPPY ENDING

One Saturday an eighteen-year-old woman entered my store in Canyon Country, California. Fortunately for both of us, I happened to be working that day. A friend had suggested she come in to see me and do the "test." The "test" is what many of our customers call the Body Language Questionnaire. I handed her the questionnaire, and she completed it at the store.

In completing the questionnaire, clients check "yes" or "no" to questions about physical ailments and conditions they may experience. These questions are arranged in sections by nutrients. The results of each section are determined by the number of *yes* answers and are categorized as *normal*, *low*, or *very low* for each nutrient. The *very low* results get immediate attention. whereas the *low* answers could indicate almost any condition. For instance, "Were they *normal* last week and are now *low*...or were they *very low* last week, and this week, through improved nutrition, they have improved to *low*?" Because a person's nutritional status can change over time, I always suggest that a person retake the questionnaire three or four times a year.

In those days, I had the nutrient deficiency analysis computer on the premises. After a customer completed the questionnaire, I was able to enter his or her answers and give the results within minutes. The computerized summary lists the spectrum of nutrients.

In the case of this eighteen-year-old, she had scored *very low* in all of the thirty-eight categories. It appeared she was deficient in every nutrient, and she was only eighteen! Perhaps these test results could be expected by someone at ninety, but not at this girl's age. This was the only time in the twenty-seven years I had given out this questionnaire that anyone had ever scored *very low* in every category! She was, according to her answers, completely deficient in everything. And her body language reflected it. With much trepidation, I handed her the test results. I then excused myself to assist another customer while she studied her outcome.

After a short while, I noticed that she had sat down and was quietly crying. When I finished with the other customer, I walked over to the young lady and asked her what was the matter. She looked at me with tears streaming down her cheeks and answered, "Look how bad I am. I'm really sick. In every area I'm *very low*. Now I see why even the doctors don't know what to do about me. Oh, I am so sick of being sick."

I needed special help with this situation, so I looked up to the heavens and asked for that special help. I said a silent thank you, and then responded, "What do you mean 'Look how bad I am?' This is one of the best questionnaires I have ever seen!"

"How can you say that?" she cried. "Every answer shows that I'm very low in everything!"

I looked right into her very red and swollen eyes and with the just-received help from above, I was able to give her a reassuring smile and say, "Yes, every answer does read *very low*, but that means only one thing."

"What?"

"It means you have reached the bottom." I paused for a moment, and then continued, "From now on, everything can only be better."

Based on the results of the questionnaire, it appeared that she was not assimilating her food—thus no energy, no enthusiasm, and a "hanging on" cold. Since the doctors couldn't find anything specifically wrong and only prescribed tranquilizers, I suggested she buy either digestive enzymes or hydrochloric acid. Hydrochloric acid is not usually indicated until a person reaches about thirty-two years of age, when the stresses of life and improper eating habits begin to cause deficiencies. This young lady had severe menstrual cramping, leg cramps, difficulty falling asleep, upper gas, lower gas, and a coated tongue. Either she wasn't getting enough minerals in her diet or she wasn't assimilating them. She claimed that she ate a lot, but the food was never digested well. She decided to try the hydrochloric acid.

Just two days later, she returned and asked if she could have a refund on her purchase. Of course I asked why. She said that when her father found out what she had bought from the vitamin store, he called the family doctor. You can only imagine what the doctor said about me, my industry, and about supplements in general!

With tears in her eyes, this young lady's last words to me as she left the store were, "I was really feeling better, a lot better. Perhaps it was all in my mind, because you took the time to care. Maybe it was the pill. After all, I did start feeling better; I mean, the food seemed to feel better in my stomach. Sometime, and I hope soon, I'll be back so that you can make me better again."

It would be nice if all of the stories in this book had happy endings. Hopefully, her story had a happy ending, even if we did not share in it firsthand.

What is the Body Language Questionnaire?

Throughout this book I have referred to a questionnaire called the Body Language Questionnaire. This consists of almost 300 questions that, when answered in the affirmative, are related to symptoms of deficiencies of vitamins, minerals, and enzymes. The questionnaire does not diagnose or prognosticate in any manner. It is used only as a tool to determine probable nutritional deficiencies. The answers are entered into a computer for evaluation. The results are printed and given to the client for an in-depth nutritional consultation. Or, if the client elects, he or she may take the results and discuss them with a doctor, nutritionist, health care counselor, or anyone else of his or her choosing.

Typical questions include: Do you have headaches, brittle fingernails, eye sensitivity to light, or a stuffy nose. A few questions would require a doctor's diagnosis. These questions would ask if you have arthritis, diabetes, or heart disease.

There is no minimum age for taking the questionnaire; however, parents would have to assist young children in answering questions.

When the questionnaire was first introduced in 1979, the suggested fee for the test results and an in-depth consultation was $25. Because Pat and I already consulted for most of our customers, without charge, we decided to offer the questionnaire for the cost of a reasonable smile. A reasonable smile. Then we would say to this sometimes hurting customer, "See, you're feeling better already."

Please visit our website at: *www.VitaminStories.com* for your "almost-free" questionnaire. Your reasonable smile will be appreciated.

If you've enjoyed the many stories in this book, then you will really appreciate Bob's second book, entitled I Found. It offers many uplifting stories based on people finding things that have, in some way, touched their lives. It is great reading and a great gift idea for that special person who might be in need of a smile or two. I Found is available by visiting: *www.CannonCorps.com* or *www.VitaminStories.com.*

Enjoy!